CW00765744

Mastering Homeopathy 3

Obstacles to Cure

Toxicity, Deficiency & Infection

Other titles by the same author:

- *Mastering Homeopathy: Accurate Daily Prescribing for a Successful Practice (2004)* ISBN 0 9752473 0 1
- *Mastering Homeopathy 2: The Treatment of Irritable Bowel Syndrome (2006)* ISBN 0 9752473 1 0
- *Treat Your Child Yourself: A Parent's Guide to Drug-Free Solutions for Common Complaints (2007)* ISBN 97809752473 2 7

In Production:
- *The Copper Children*
- *Treat Your Self*

Mastering Homeopathy 3

Obstacles to Cure

Toxicity, Deficiency & Infection

A Practitioner's Manual

Jon Gamble
BA ND Adv Dip Hom

Series Editor
Nyema Hermiston
RN ND Adv Dip Hom

***K**aruna* **Publishing**
2010

First published in Australia by
Karuna Publishing
122 Church Street
Wollongong NSW 2500
karuna@bigpond.net.au

© Jon Gamble 2010
Reprinted 2011
All rights reserved. No part of this book may be reproduced, stored in a retrieval system, or transmitted in any form or by any means, electronic, mechanical or otherwise, without the prior written permission of the author.

Every effort has been made to ensure that this book is free from error or omissions. However, the author and publishers shall not accept responsibility for injury, loss or damage occasioned to any person acting or refraining from action as a result of material in this book whether or not such injury, loss or damage is in any way due to any negligent act or omission, breach of duty or default on the part of the author or publishers.

This book is not intended to replace competent medical advice nor should the recommendations herein be relied upon as representing every possible presentation of an illness. The differential diagnoses should not be construed as exhaustive. The therapeutic recommendations are provided as treatment examples only. This work is largely the result of clinical observations and is intended only for fully trained health care practitioners.

National Library of Australia Cataloguing-in-Publication entry

Author:	Gamble, Jon, 1959-
Title:	Obstacles to cure: treating toxicity, deficiency and infection / Jon Gamble.
ISBN:	9780975247334 (special limited edition reprint)
Series:	Mastering homeopathy; 3.
Notes:	Includes bibliographical references and index.
Subjects:	Chronic diseases--Treatment--Handbooks, manuals, etc.
	Chronically ill--Care.
	Heavy metals--Toxicology.
	Malnutrition--Treatment--Handbooks, manuals, etc.
	Deficiency diseases--Treatment--Handbooks, manuals, etc.
	Infection--Treatment--Handbooks, manuals, etc.
	Homeopathy--Handbooks, manuals, etc.

Dewey Number: 616.044
Printed in Australia by Griffin Press
Cover design by Tina Mulholland

Foreword

Working as a homeopath or any kind of complementary health care practitioner in Australia in the year 2010 requires a far more mindful, educated and possibly even more cautious approach than what it did 20 years ago. For this reason, the release of Jon's book is significantly timely and of value.

Homeopathy has always been something of a soft target for skeptics because there is so much material for them to criticise – everything from the high dilutions of the remedies and the premise that 'less is more', to the even more difficult concept of 'like cures like'. Much of the world uses the western model of medicine and many find it difficult to believe that such dilute medicines can be effective or curative.

However, it is not only the homeopathic model which faces difficulty in Australia. During 2003, the whole of the complementary medicine industry in Australia faced a substantial blow to its credibility when the Therapeutic Goods Administration (TGA) created unnecessary chaos amongst consumers and retailers alike by recalling 1500 natural products under a Class-one recall (Class –one signifying "imminent danger of death"). As a consequence of these events and possibly as a result of global demands for 'proof' as a basis to endorse credibility, there are strong drives towards using more 'science based' methods to support diagnosis and prescriptions. Patients have become more informed and are more discerning. Information is available on every subject at the touch of a computer key and society is more litigious than ever.

In this climate, practitioners need to be better informed about options for their patients, better educated about the 'tools' available to them and more accepting of the fact that they are accountable for their advice (or lack of advice) to their clients.

Jon's book is a gift to those practitioners who enjoy the benefits of being informed and who have a desire to get to the root of their patient's ill health. It contains a treasure house of information, not only about tests and obstacles to cure, but also about remedies and which potency is more efficient to use than others and how long it should be used for.The style of writing is clear and easy to follow with many good case examples and there are wonderful reminders about the importance of common sense, the dangers of jumping to conclusions and the value of being cautious and practical. I believe the information Jon has put together will inspire practitioners to broaden their case taking criteria. It will also help them to identify what they are dealing with, to understand what the implications for their patients are, and it will educate them on how to formulate a responsible plan of action. The book is concise and well written and should be of enormous value to any complementary healthcare practitioner.

Maryanne Logan: President of the *Australian Homeopathic Association* (NSW)

Dedication

To the memory of Dr Garry Gow

Friend and Colleague

Contents

PART 4 Case Studies

Preface

Many people have played a part in the manifestation of this book. All the patients upon whom we have attempted new treatment protocols and unusual remedies deserve our thanks. Some of our 'Eureka' moments have arisen from these experiments, while others have come to nothing. This book contains the results of our Eureka moments. We have written here the methods and protocols which work for most people most of the time. We have described some of the common reasons why our chosen remedies do not work and what to do about them.

In this preface I am using the 'we', whereas in the rest of the book I use 'I'. That is because I here wish to acknowledge all the hidden work contributed by Nyema Hermiston. Nyema has again edited the book within an inch of its life. She has provided much of the background research and thoroughly revised each chapter. The chapter on Nutritional Deficiency is Nyema's progeny. The writing of a book is only one small part of its creation. That writing necessarily has to arise out of hours of discussion and workshopping. Then there is the tossing around of ideas with reference to clinical feedback. Those ideas have to be knitted together into a workable and useful whole without which they remain unusable strands of thread. Nyema has played a major role in all these aspects and the creation of this work lies in her hands as well as my own. I however, accept the responsibility for any errors that may become apparent in time.

I would also like to acknowledge the draft comments made by two of my colleagues: Linda Beaver and Christine Pope.

Jon Gamble
September 2010

Introduction

Few would argue that the application of the *simillimum* leads to a rapid resolution of symptoms. When the correct homeopathic medicine, or '*simillimum*' is applied, the cure is profound. As homeopaths, we have all seen profound transformations in patients. Sometimes they are our own patients, other times we learn about amazing cures from our colleagues.

There are also many patients, in homeopathic parlance, who are 'non responders.' Even in the face of this, many practitioners believe that applying the *simillimum* is all that is necessary in the day-to-day treatment of our patients.

The subject of this book is *not* about patients who respond brilliantly to the *similimum*; it is about those patients who, despite repeated application of the best-selected homeopathic remedies, do not respond to treatment.

As a homeopath, it is easy to believe that, when a patient has not responded to well selected remedies, that you just have to dig deeper, treat the *miasm*, give Sulphur, and so on. But what if the non-responsiveness is due to a toxic or infective agent, or due to ongoing and unrecognised chemical exposure? Clinical experience made me aware of a growing accumulation of toxic, infective and chemical agents that need to be removed or excluded from the patient's environment before they can recover. A simple example of this is mercury toxicity from dental amalgams, in a patient who had been trying (classically prescribed) homeopathic remedies for over a decade, yet did not start to recover from Chronic Fatigue Syndrome until her mercury amalgams were removed. Once this 'obstacle to cure' was identified, treatment was focussed on removing the mercury toxicity and the patient responded to treatment for the first time in many years.

Heavy metal toxicity is common and its removal is essential. Identifying it with Hair Tissue Mineral Analysis has led to greater clarity and better results in my practice.

In the context of the huge increase of toxic exposures to which the human race has been exposed since World War I, this book explores the increasing *unlikelihood* of the homeopath's ability to deal with all aspects of our patients' health using traditional homeopathic prescribing alone. Therefore, I would like to share the tools which I have found useful for dealing with 21st century health issues.

I have come to the conclusion that the homeopath's toolbox must contain a *range of tools*, because patient presentations vary so much. From one case to the next we have to develop a flexible approach to choosing the best tools needed to treat the case before us. Every methodology has value provided it can produce the desired result for patient and practitioner. The *patient is completely unconcerned* with which methodology is used: his or her only concern is with the outcome: to be free from their complaint. Usually, this complaint has been present for some time, often years, before patients come to a homeopathic clinic, so it is usually safe to assume that you have a chronic case sitting in front of you.

History has shown that there are numerous methods at our disposal in the use of homeopathic medicines:
- *Boenninghausen method*
- *Bowel nosodes*
- *Central delusion of the patient.*
- *Colour*
- *Classical approach*
- *Essence of the patient*
- *Facial diagnosis*
- *Gemmotherapy*
- *Hahnemannian*
- *Isopathy*
- *Kentian*
- *Mineral therapy*
- *Organ drainage*
- *Sequential approach*
- *Tautopathy*
- *Therapeutics / Clinical homeopathy*
- *Totality of symptoms*
- *Vital sensation.*

There are always instances where one adheres to the 'classical' approach of 'treat the patient, not the disease', which is just one of the methods available. The *patient's response* will tell you if it was an appropriate choice. It is a testament to the challenge of finding the appropriate medicine that so many techniques have been developed. It is worth remembering that Kent's *Repertory* contained vastly more physical than mental symptoms. Experience tells me that it is a folly to ignore (or downgrade in importance) the physical presentation of symptoms common to a disease, since every symptom presentation is an individual response to that disease. Individual responses are the quintessential markers of homeopathic prescribing.

The original homeopaths, mostly doctors, had to diagnose their patients. They needed to do this to understand their patient's disease. Lay homeopaths may have fewer diagnostic tools at their disposal to find out what disease a patient has but it makes it no less important. How are we to address the illness if we do not know what it is?

It is easy to announce one's remarkable results to other practitioners – we all have them. For ten years I believed if only I could develop enough skill to perceive the internal world of the patient, I could find the *simillimum*. I wrote up my successful cases and in hindsight, I probably gave the impression that these successes were a fair representation of my practice. But actually they weren't. The amazing successes were the *exceptions* to my practice. I recorded far more failures than successes. To keep practising homeopathy, flying solo amongst difficult odds, I had to keep believing in the ultimate cure using the *simillimum*. If you do not keep believing in it, and most of your cases do not succeed, you stop practising because it is not sustainable financially, ethically or personally.

After ten years I very nearly went out of practice.

My turning point was when this 45-year-old man presented with diarrhoea that was worse before any event. He was claustrophobic and craved sugar. Anticipatory diarrhoea with claustrophobia and sugar cravings? Easy! Of course, I gave him *Argentum nitricum*. Several potencies of *Argentum nitricum* later, he had not improved. This was my end of the road! After ten years, how could I have confidence in my method and my tools (homeopathy) when such a clear case failed to respond to the indicated remedy? It was hair-pulling frustration! Give me a reason to stay in this job!

I didn't know then, but I know now, *why* the remedy did not work, even though the patient may have been a textbook *Argentum nitricum*. I knew *who* I was treating but I did not know *what* I was treating. The single methodology which I had struggled to use for ten years excluded '*what*' the patient was suffering from and only focussed on '*who*' was suffering from it. Repertorising the case did not reveal a successful remedy.

As it turned out, this patient had chronic gut parasites. He did not know it. His doctor did not know it and I did not know it either. As homeopaths, we might never think of it with this presentation. If the patient has been seeing their doctor for some time, it is easy to assume, 'that has already been checked out before seeing me...'.

What I learned from this was to ask *why* the patient had these symptoms. What would cause this man's symptoms? If he was truly a constitutional *Argentum nitricum*, how come his symptoms only appeared now, later in his life – why did he not have them all his life? What would cause this patient's symptoms? Will *Argentum nitricum* get rid of parasites? In this case: no. I tried several potencies all to no avail. This patient needed *Cina*. I have come to find that parasites cause a disparate symptom picture, which is often unrelated to the patient's constitutional medicine. The symptom picture exists *despite* the constitutional aspects of the patient, not because of them. Gut parasites can be an obstacle to cure. Since this case I have treated many patients with *Cina* instead of their constitutional remedy with great success.

It is not easy to change your methodology to deal with cases that do not respond and find a different approach to apply. After 23 years of practice now, I have found that finding a *cause* for the presenting problem diagnosis and any *obstacle to cure* is equally important to understanding the mental state. There are times when the mental state can be *caused by* the physical problem: for which I give examples later.

My practice has never been so exciting. My patients have never been better. The great news is that what Hahnemann wrote 200 years ago on understanding what is to be treated is just as relevant, perhaps more relevant, now.

I hope that you will find this book a useful addition to your practice and that it will help you to solve some of your obstinate cases. With such high criticism of homeopathy in the press it is in everyone's best interests to expand their skills and successfully treat our patients.

Three broad areas of obstacles to cure are discussed in this book:

Part 1: Deficiency
- Nutritional Deficiency in Chapter 2.

Part 2: Infection
- Viral, bacterial and other infections in Chapter 3.

Part 3: Toxicity
- Heavy Metals in Chapters 4 and 5.
- Chemicals in Chapter 6.
- Iatrogenic disease in Chapter 7.

Part 4: Cases
Case examples of each of these obstacles to cure.

For practitioners who are not familiar with Hair Tissue Mineral Analysis, I recommend reading Appendix 1 and 2 before reading Chapters 4, 5 and 9.

Chapter 1
Discovering the Underpinning Cause of Disease

In this beginning chapter, I would like to outline the work that I do and how I came to do it. It has been a long process of weaving in and out of homeopathic philosophy, having what I considered too many failed cases. Over the years, I have developed my own prescribing system, which has a strong clinical approach, with the emphasis being on treating the fundamental cause of disease. This cause may be a previous illness, a nutritional deficiency, a *miasm*, or, as you will see, environmental toxicity. When I look back, I see so many instances where my homeopathic education has been an impediment to seeing this fundamental cause clearly, without 'transcendental speculations', to use Hahnemann's words. Over time, I started to penetrate those previously insurmountable cases. I hope that I can describe to you what I do so that you can also use it.

In practice, we take the case and select a homeopathic remedy based on our chosen methodology. Some patients respond well and some do not. With more experience, our prescribing skills improve and more patients benefit from our treatment. But there are a growing number of patients who do not respond to any treatment. If we are lucky, these patients will persist with their treatment so that we can eventually find success. When my patients present with intractable health issues that simply do not respond to the well-selected remedy, I ask myself:

Have I chosen an incorrect remedy?

Have I come up against an obstacle to cure? If so, what is that obstacle?

These questions and some solutions that I have found to them are the topic of this book.

I have come to realise that obstacles to cure are many and bring new meaning to the concept of *miasms*. Obstacles to cure, as you will see, include simple nutritional deficiencies, infections and man-made synthetic chemicals and heavy metals. For a long time though, my most common obstacle to cure lay within me: my case analysis. I did not understand what Hahnemann boldly announces on the first page of his *Organon*, in Aphorisms 3 to 5: *one must correctly recognise the fundamental cause of disease before choosing a remedy*. Blinded by the philosophy of prescribing on the 'totality of symptoms', sadly for my patients, it took many years for me to change the focus from adhering to this philosophy to practising what Hahnemann was telling us:

§ 3 *Clearly perceive what* is to be cured (ie knowledge of diseases). This includes awareness of the obstacles to recovery and how to remove them.

§ 4 Be aware of *causes* of disease (ie pathophysiology)

§ 5 Determine the exciting (acute) and fundamental causes (chronic) due to miasms (ie obstacles to cure)

Now I would like to go through each of the following points and describe how I endeavour to use the wisdom of these aphorisms in my practice.

---

1. Identify what is to be cured (§§3-4)
Look for the fundamental cause of the presenting complaint before considering which remedy to prescribe.

2. Recognise any obstacles to cure (§3-5)

3. Choose the most appropriate remedy (§3)

---

1. Identify what is to be cured (Org §§3-4)
Look for the fundamental cause of the presenting complaint before considering which remedy to prescribe.

It is a familiar story for any practitioner: everyone has cases which:
- Do not respond to the well indicated remedy
- Respond well for a time but then relapse
- Partially respond, some symptoms persist or new symptoms appear.

In response, do we choose another remedy? How do we choose this remedy, and upon what do we base it? Do we retake the case?
When a prescription is repeatedly unsuccessful, my question becomes: *What is the pathophysiology in this case?*

Example

A woman has difficulty swallowing. She describes the sensation of a lump in her throat and is feeling quite anxious about it. A death in her family several months ago preceded this symptom.

Repertorisation:
-Throat, lump, plug, sensation in
   -Grief, after
   -Hysterical
-Aliments, grief, after

I decide this patient has globus hystericus, caused by grief and anxiety, and prescribe Ignatia.
Ignatia fails.

At the next consultation I discover that there is a rising sensation, so I choose Moschus, another of the 'hysteric' remedies.

Moschus fails. Next I try Asafoetida. This also fails.

Discussion
By the third unsuccessful prescription, the patient stops seeing me. I have lost the case.

Let us start again. Before repertorising the case, we will consider *what is to be treated, not who is to be treated.* The question to ask in this case is *why* can't this person swallow? What are the differential diagnoses?

Am I treating:
• Bulbar palsy
• Foreign body
• Gastric reflux
• Globus hystericus
• Goitre
• Scleroderma of the throat
• Tonsillitis
• Tumour?

Here are four possible scenarios for this case:

a) The patient returns with the same symptoms, having had a gastroscopy. The diagnosis is scleroderma of the throat. The mucous membrane has become hard and tight, giving her a sensation of a lump, and there is difficult swallowing. The 'sensation' is more than subjective, it has a physical pathology. Given the severity of this diagnosis, and the dreadful feeling she must have in her throat, her anxiety is not surprising. Now the symptom of anxiety is not so strong in the repertorisation because it is a normal response to this illness, for which there is no medical cure.

To the rubrics chosen above, I add:
-Skin, scleroderma

Whichever remedy I choose, it has to include this rubric. We might say this is the most important rubric – even though it is only a 'particular'. The remedy choices are now narrowed down to *Calcarea carb, Graphites* and *Hydrocotle*.

b) The patient returns with a diagnosis of goitre from hypothyroidism. Again, the 'sensation' is more than just a sensation, there is a physical pathology. Anxiety is a common symptom of thyroid disturbance, so it does not carry as much weight as I first thought. Now I add the rubric:
-Glands, thyroid, goitre
   -Constriction, with
I have narrowed the remedy choice to: Calcarea sulph, CROTALIS C, Iodum, Lycopodium and Spongia. Again this 'particulars' rubric is vital.

c) Gastroscopy has revealed silent gastro-oesophageal reflux. I add

-Stomach, Lump, plug, sensation of, oesophagus

The remedy choices are: Allium c, Causticum, Coccus cacti, Conium, Gelsemium, Lobelia, Plumbum or Pulsatilla. The 'particulars' rubric is again vital.

d) Gastroscopy reveals that the patient has throat cancer.

Identifying the cause of the symptoms (*what specifically is to be treated*) changes the rubrics I choose and therefore the list of remedy possibilities. *The symptoms must make pathophysiological sense.* Knowing *what* I am treating, must influence the treatment I choose. Making the wrong pathophysiological diagnosis severely limits the likelihood of successfully treating a case.

The 'cause', as Hahnemann clearly states in §6, must be *free from 'transcendental speculations'*. In the case above, it is easy to assume that the cause of the symptoms was recent grief or shock.

Much homeopathic education emphasises finding the patient's 'constitutional medicine', analysing all of which can achieve brilliant results, but *only if they address the undepinning cause of the presenting symptoms.*

The patient is much more than a mere collection of disparate symptoms. If one chooses to look for the most appropriate remedy for the patient before identifying the most likely cause for the problem, the likelihood of a successful prescription is reduced.

Aphorism 3 on the first page of the *Organon* makes this clear (bold print is my emphasis):

§3 If the physician clearly perceives what is to be cured in diseases, that is to say, in every individual case of disease (*knowledge of disease, indication*), if he clearly perceives what is curative in medicines, that is to say, in each individual medicine (*knowledge of medicinal powers*), **and if he knows how to adapt, according to clearly defined principles, what is curative in medicines to what he has discovered to be undoubtedly morbid in the patient,** so that the recovery must ensure – **to adapt it, as well in respect to the suitability of the medicine most appropriate according to its mode of action to the case before him** (*choice of remedy, the medicine indicated*), as also in respect to the exact mode of preparation and quantity of it required (proper *dose*), and the proper period for repeating the dose:- if finally, he **knows the *obstacles to recovery* in each case and is aware how to remove them,** so that the restoration may be permanent: *then he understands how to treat judiciously and rationally, and he is a true practitioner of the healing art.*

§4 He is likewise a preserver of health if he knows the *things that derange and cause disease, and how to remove them from persons in health.*[1]

Hahnemann is asking us to determine the *fundamental cause, which* can be objectively verified. When that has been determined, he asks us to adapt what we know of *materia medica* to meet the fundamental disease cause. 'Adapt' is a very precise word. Hahnemann is bestowing great confidence in our ability to use his method in an individual way. Yet he is very clear when he tells us we must *know the fundamental cause before we individualise the case (what we are treating comes before who we are treating).* If the fundamental cause is an obstacle, then we will soon find out when the usual application of the *similimum* fails. So the next task is to identify that obstacle.

2. Recognise any obstacles to cure (§§3-5)

Let us revisit Aphorism 5:

§5 Useful to the physician in assisting him to cure are the particulars of the most probable *exciting cause* of the acute disease, as also the most significant points in the whole history of the chronic disease, to enable him to discover its *fundamental cause*, which is generally due to a chronic miasm. In these investigations, the ascertainable physical constitution of the patient, (especially when the disease is chronic) his moral and intellectual character, his occupation, mode of living and habits, his social and domestic relations, his age, sexual function &c., are to be taken into consideration.

Successful patient outcomes require us to remove our homeopathic hats entirely when we take the case. Analysing the case asks much more of us than toting up the symptoms. It also requires us at times to step outside of our preferred methodology. Homeopathic analysis must come *after* having taken the case and pencilled in possible causations.

During case taking, we need two things, neither of which have anything to do with choosing a homeopathic medicine. First, to create an empathic space in whatever way we can. Entering the patient's world by listening to and getting a feel for the way they describe their suffering. How does this patient make me feel when he is in my room? Do I feel angry, sad, anxious? That is most likely how the patient feels. If the patient is not feeling sad, having narrated his sad story, then why not? Does it all make sense? What disease phenomenon, mental, physical or emotional, may cause this? This is what Hahnemann says in Aphorism 3:

---

[1] Hahnemann, Dr S, *Organon of Medicine, 5th & 6th eds, translated* by R Dudgeon, B Jain Publishers, New Delhi, 1990 ed.

§3 (extract) *and if he knows how to adapt,* according to clearly defined principles, what is curative in medicines to *what he has discovered to be undoubtedly morbid in the patient,*

Once the empathic interchange has taken place it is time to put on the thinking cap – but not the homeopathic cap - yet. *The symptoms have to make sense in terms of pathophysiology.* If someone has difficulty swallowing with a sensation of a lump in the throat, we have to make sure we rule out the physical pathologies before we jump in with a speculative hypothesis. We first need differential diagnoses of what can be causing these symptoms:

Think expansively: what disease could be causing these sets of symptoms?
- Anxiety?
- Nutritional deficiency? (common)
- Some kind of toxicity?
- Thyroid disturbance?
- Viral infection?

Example
Woman with Chronic Back Pain
This 25 year-old woman with back pain had tried it all – osteopathy, homeopathy, pain management and so on. Her pain was unusual – she had burning, shooting, tingling pain with paraesthesia. None of the usual therapies, including homeopathy, had been effective. One might expect these symptoms in the leg (sciatica), yet if felt in the back, are unusual. In fact, they suggest a transient neuritis or neuralgia. As I reflected on this, the symptoms reminded me of shingles. When I looked into her history, it revealed her pain was preceded by a transient vesicular eruption on her back at the site of the pain. What seemed like a musculoskeletal problem had all the hallmarks of post-zoster neuralgia!

No one was surprised more than I, when after eight weeks of Arsenicum *and* Herpes Zoster Nosode, *her pain had completely disappeared. In the end, it was necessary to treat the cause of her pain, not just prescribe on the totality of her presenting symptoms.*

Case scenario
The patient suffers from ongoing headaches. Possible causes are:

- Brain Tumour (unlikely, but not impossible)
- Dehydration
- Eyestrain
- Food sensitivity
- Hypoglycaemia
- Neck misalignment
- Stress
- Sinus or gum infection.

Each of these causes involves a different body system and would therefore require a very different repertorisation resulting in a different homeopathic (or lifestyle) prescription.

Simple observation of the patient can clarify the origin of the problem.

Patient examination
The course of a consultation affords ample opportunity to gather simple information about our patients. Palpation and observation may tell us more than the patient can. Abdominal pain can be caused by faecal impaction, which is clearly palpable. Ear discomfort may be a fungal infection, otitis media, or neither. Otoscopy will reveal this. A joint may feel hot, puffy or cold.

Other examples:
1. A 10 year-old boy had pain in his left ear only when he swallowed. There was no fever. Otoscopic exam showed a normal canal and tympanum. Examination of his submandibular glands showed marked hypertrophy with some tenderness. He had green nasal catarrh and the next day he developed conjunctivitis. This boy had developed a mild head cold with conjunctivitis and lymphatic congestion, but there was no involvement of the middle ear. Only examination helped to exclude otitis media.

2. When a patient has a chest complaint, check for abnormal chest sounds! This case was a real eye-opener.
An 18 year-old male had breathing distress for two days. His chest sounds were normal. In asthma, pneumonia or bronchitis you would hear altered chest sounds, so I referred him for medical assessment. On his chest x-ray, a mediastinal carcinoma was found.

The three broad areas of obstacle to cure discussed here are:

Nutritional deficiency

Nutritional deficiency is common in the developed world, and is the topic of Chapter 2. Deficiencies that I see repeatedly in my clinics are zinc, magnesium, iodine and iron.

Infection
Since Hahnemann's *Chronic Diseases,* the idea that organisms cause disease is fundamental to homeopathic philosophy and treatment. He enunciated this clearly in the four *miasms*:

- Psoric (scabies) Sarcoptes scabiei
- Sycotic (gonorrhoea) *Neisseria gonorrhoeae*
- Syphilitic (syphilis) *Treponema pallidum*
- Tubercular (Tuberculosis) organism *Mycobacterium tuberculosis.*

The term *miasm* is a Greek word meaning 'to pollute'. With the benefit of microbiology, far more organisms (*miasms*) have been identified as pathogenic, including the ability of some microbes to cause mental illness. It should come as no surprise to homeopaths that microbes can cause profound mental disturbance. This brings a far wider view of the notion of illness being caused by one or more of the four *miasms*.

Treating bacterial, viral and parasitic infection is a fundamental part of any homeopathic practice. Among these are Lyme Disease, PANDAS (Paediatric Autoimmune Neuropsychiatric Disorder Associated with Streptococcus) and all the viruses that were unrecognised in the 19th century. Many recognisable viruses are responsible for a wide range of illnesses that, unless addressed, amount to obstacles to a patient's recovery. Some of these are glandular fever (Epstein Barr virus) and herpes viruses, well known for affecting the nervous system.

Toxicity
Toxicity was of course a problem 200 years ago, with heavy metals such as mercury used as treatment for syphilis and arsenic as a panacea for every ill in the form of Fowlers solution, used widely from the 1800's to the 1930's.[2]

With the advent of the mining and petrochemical industries, there are now many more obstacles to cure that did not exist in the 19th century. This requires of us to build on the foundational premise of the *miasms*.

Some of our new disease-producing challenges are:

Chemicals
- Organochloride and organophosphate pesticides and herbicides
- Environmental xenoestrogens.

Heavy Metals
Cadmium, lead, mercury and other metals (heavy metal toxicity) can now easily be identified in some unresponsive patients, via hair tissue mineral analysis.

Iatrogenesis
- More widespread iatrogenic disease, including vaccine damage.

---

3. *Finally*, choose the most appropriate remedy (§3)
by reference to the most striking, rare and peculiar symptoms of the patient (case individualisation).

§6 *'...the futility of transcendental speculations...'*
The unprejudiced observer – well aware of the *futility of transcendental speculations* which can receive no confirmation from experience – be his powers of penetration ever so great, takes not of nothing in every individual disease, except the changes in the health of the body and of the

---

[2]Allen, W, *War on Bugs*, **ISBN**-13: 978-1933392462

mind (morbid phenomena, accidents, symptoms), which can be perceived externally by means of the senses; that is to say, he notices only the deviations from the former healthy state of the now diseased individual, which are felt by the patient himself, remarked by those around him and observed by the physician. All these perceptible signs represent the disease in its whole extent, that is, together they form the true and only conceivable portrait of the disease.[3]

Now that we have decided the fundamental cause of the patient's symptoms, it is time to decide a treatment plan, which often, but not always, requires choosing the most appropriate homeopathic medicine. *This* is the time to take the individual generals and particulars into account, *provided that your diagnosis is retained in the case analysis*. This way of case taking turns things around the other way: we decide on the 'what' *before* we treat the 'who'.

In regard to the patient with difficult swallowing and a sense of constriction, if there is a goitre, this must be included in the case analysis and remedy selection. If we do not know the fundamental cause, it is necessary to consider one or more differential diagnoses. Using the same case example, if there were other symptoms of hypothyroidism (eg hair loss and weight gain) then it would be reasonable to make a provisional diagnosis of goitre, pending a pathology test. In any case, once a diagnosis is made, *only then* is it time to put on the homeopathic hat.

There is nothing new in this premise. Many practitioners have described the importance of knowing accurate diagnosis (§§3-5). Practitioners who have done substantial work in this area are:
- o Dr Jean Elmiger showed us how to locate and antidote the disease effects which have negatively impacted the patient (what has become known as sequential treatment)[4].
- o The late Dr Tinus Smits has shown us how to antidote vaccine damage. [5]

Treatment approaches in this book include:
- Nutritional supplementation
- Homeopathic medicine – applying the similimum
- Tautopathic medicine[6]
- Isopathy.

---

[3] Hahnemann Dr S *Organon of Medicine, 5th & 6th eds, translated* by R Dudgeon B Jain Publishers, New Delhi, 1990 ed.
[4] Elmiger, Dr J, *Rediscovering Real Medicine: New Horizons in Homeopathy*, Vega, London, 2001
[5] Smits, Dr T, http://www.post-vaccination-syndrome.com/3890/treatment.aspx
[6] Tautopathy refers to isopathic treatment using potentised preparations of chemicals, which includes allopathic drugs, industrial chemicals, pesticides and household chemicals *source:* Swayne, J, *International Dictionary of Homeopathy*, Churchill Livingstone, 2000

Chapter 2
Nutritional Deficiencies and Imbalances

§3 [I]f finally, he knows the obstacles to recovery in each case and is aware how to remove them, so that the restoration may be permanent: then he understands how to treat judiciously and rationally, and he is a true practitioner of the healing art.

§5 [A]lso the most significant points in the whole history of the chronic disease, to enable him to discover its fundamental cause which is generally due to a chronic miasm. In these investigations, the ascertainable physical constitution of the patient (especially when the disease is chronic) his moral and intellectual character, *his occupation, mode of living and habits,* his social and domestic relations, his age, sexual function, &c., are to be taken into consideration.

In Aphorism 5, Hahnemann is describing what is now called 'lifestyle' of which diet is a part. It is common in practice for some patients, often children, to have diets that are nutritionally poor, highly processed, sugary diets. Sometimes, improving diet can improve health to an extraordinary degree. Without proper nutrition, how can we expect our patients to improve using the selected medicine alone? Here are two case examples to demonstrate this point – one that received no homeopathic medicine and one that did.

Example
A woman in her late 60's with life-long asthma presented for relief of her symptoms. She looked extremely unhealthy, was wheezing and breathless. She had been taking Prednisone for decades, and her case was a myriad of acute and chronic symptoms that made for a prescribing nightmare. Where to start?

She said she just wanted to get healthy enough to go on an overseas trip. Her nutrition was almost certainly compromised due to the years of cortico-steriods, so I prescribed a high dose vitamin and mineral formula.

The next time she contacted the clinic was after her overseas trip, wanting another bottle of "those pills". She phoned every couple of months for another "bottle of pills" for several years. Her quality of life had been improved with a simple nutritional supplementation. She did not need another consultation, because she was so happy with her health and so I never prescribed her a homeopathic remedy.

Prolonged use of cortico-steroids depletes mineral absorption, particularly calcium, and causes osteoporosis.[7] Will the correct homeopathic remedy address a nutritional deficiency caused by medication? In this case, the obstacle to cure was addressed well by a nutritional supplement. A homeopathic medicine should provide at least this much improvement to justify using it alone, without addressing obvious nutritional issues.

If a patient's nutritional status is compromised, well-selected homeopathic medicines may sometimes be ineffective, as shown by this case:

A two-year-old girl with frequent viral infections had had a range of homeopathic remedies for her repeated infections over several months, including Calcarea phos. She had a pasty complexion and a poor appetite. It was unclear why she was not responding to homeopathic medicines, until I prescribed an iron supplement. At her follow up, even before her mother started to speak, it was easy to tell she had improved, because I could see her rosy cheeks. Since receiving the iron supplement, her appetite had improved, she was much healthier, had better colour and recovered from the infections more quickly. Iron deficiency anaemia[8] was this girl's obstacle to cure.

Nutritional deficiency is an easily overlooked and common obstacle to cure even in contemporary practice. It is useful to become aware of the conditions that specific nutritional deficiencies can cause.

This chapter is divided into two parts: *nutritional deficiency* and *nutritional imbalance*. It explores *some* nutritional deficiencies that commonly present in my clinic. It is not an exhaustive list of conditions caused by nutritional deficiencies, rather those that I have been found to be 'obstacles to cure' in a homeopathic context.

Some reasons for nutritional deficiency:
- Cancer
- Constitutional weakness
- Heavy metal toxicity
- Mineral imbalance
- Poor diet
- Poor gut function and malabsorption; Crohn's disease, Coeliac disease
- Side effects of medications (eg *cortico-steroids*).

When taking the case, checking the patient's appetite and diet may give us vital information about nutritional deficiency. Most would agree that a homeopathic medicine has the capacity to enhance mineral absorption, but it is unlikely to be a substitute for frank deficiency.

---

[7] Sambrook, P, "Corticosteroid osteoporosis" Best Pract Res Clin Rheumatol. 2001 Jul; 15(3): 401-13. http://www.ncbi.nlm.nih.gov/pubmed/11485337

[8] Most children do not have their haemaglobin tested unless they become seriously ill.

Assessing Nutrition

First, knowledge of conditions caused by deficiency, such as iron deficiency anemia, is essential and referral for testing is an important part of any practice. In addition to blood test one can also use Hair Tissue Mineral Analysis (HTMA) which gives a wider perspective about mineral uptake. An orientation of HTMA is given in Appendix 2.

Common Nutritional Deficiencies

Iodine

Iodine deficiency disorder (IDD) is the leading global cause of preventable mental defect. According to the latest estimates from the World Health Organisation, close to two billion of the world's population are affected by IDD.[9] Even in developed countries, moderate to severe iodine deficiency can cause up to a 15 point IQ loss causing a loss of gifted people in the community. See the table below.

Percentage of (Randomly Selected) **Populations with Mild-Severe Iodine Deficiency Disorder**[10]

Australia	46.3	Malaysia	57
Canada	0	Netherlands	37.5
China	15.7	New Zealand	0
Cuba	51	Norway	0
Denmark	70.8	Poland	64
France	60.4	Spain	50
Germany	27	Sweden	0
India	31.3	Switzerland	50
Ireland	60.8	UK	0
Italy	55	USA	19.4
Japan	0		

The work in Tibet of Professor Cres Eastman, Regional Coordinator of International Council for the Control of Iodine Deficiency[11], has earned him the title 'the man who saved a million brains.' However, there is a grisly twist to this story. Professor Eastman, now coordinator of the Institute of Clinical Pathology and Medical Research at Westmead Hospital in Sydney, has tested Australian children's iodine levels[12] to find that far away from Tibet, in well-nourished Australia, some 50 per cent of the children he tested were found to be iodine deficient.

---

[9] www.WHO.int/
[10] International Council for the Control of Iodine Deficiency Disorders
http://www.iccidd.org/media/IodineNetworkScorecard2010.pdf

[11] http://www.iccidd.org/pages/contact.php
[12] Are Australian children iodine deficient? Australian National Iodine Nutrition Study Results.
http://www.mja.com.au/public/issues/184_04_200206/li10728_fm.html

In Australia, dietary iodine was once unwittingly acquired from milk, through 'accidental positive contamination', when dairy equipment was sterilised using iodine. In the past ten years or so, iodine has been replaced by a chlorine-based steriliser, leaving the Australian population, again unwittingly, without iodine in its food supply. To address this problem, iodine is now being added to non-organic bread in some states.

We think of iodine as being associated with thyroid function. While this is true, the thyroid only holds 31% of the body's iodine. In iodine deficiency, the thyroid competes with other body tissue for the available iodine and the other body tissues suffer first. Iodine deficiency has been implicated in polycystic ovarian disease, fibrocystic breast disease and in some forms of cancer. Japan has the lowest incidence of cancer in the western world (with the exception of bowel cancer) and one thought is that this is due to their good iodine stores from the high consumption of seaweed in Japanese diet.

Natural treatment of cystic conditions and cancer often includes iodine supplementation. It is also well documented that iodine deficiency is linked with ADHD and other learning difficulties.

Symptoms of iodine deficiency
- Cystic hypertrophy of endocrine or reproductive glands (goitre; fibrocystic breast disease, etc)
- Developmental delay
- Learning and behavioural disorders
- Mental retardation
- Thyroid disorders.

Causes of Iodine Deficiency
- Brominated vegetable oil (bromide) also found in soft drinks
- Dietary deficiency
- Fluoride (fluorine competes with iodine)[13]
- Goitrogens (inhibiting iodine activity are in foods such as cabbage, broccoli, turnip, cauliflower, plus soybean).[14]

Testing iodine levels
Iodine levels can be measured by an inexpensive urine test, which in Australia, is available through Medicare. Less accurate, but as a guide, is a skin patch test. There are several methods, but one is to put two drops of iodine on a sensitive skin area such as inside the arm and allow it to dry. If the deep yellow colour of the iodine disappears quickly, deficiency is indicated. If the colour is still present eight hours later, then deficiency is less likely. In clinic, this can offer an initial guide to iodine levels.

It is important to assess iodine levels in all thyroid disorders, ovarian and breast cysts and children with learning and behavioural disorders. Iodine

---

[13] Patients with thyroid disorders should avoid drinking fluoridated water since fluoride is a known endocrine disruptor.
[14] Gaitan, E, 'Goitrogens in Food and Water', *Annual Review of Nutrition,* 1990; 10: 21-39

replacement can result in an improvement in a patient's symptoms, where homeopathic medicine may not. If iodine deficiency is present in your patient, it stands as an obstacle to cure until corrected. With the amount of deficiency in 'well nourished' patients, the case for iodine levels screening at birth or soon afterwards is strong, and would be a significant preventive public health care strategy.

Sources of Iodine
The best natural sources of iodine are from the seabed, particularly seaweed (kelp). Iodised salt on food and in cooking is a reliable source. Many nutritional supplements contain iodine and there are several of specific iodine supplements available.

Iron
Iron deficiency anaemia is surprisingly common, not only in menstruating women, but in children under the age of 2 years. Since the demands on the body's iron stores are greater during bacterial infections, it is important to check for iron deficiency in patients who have recurring, or have just recovered from, such infections. Due to dietary trends, many families eat little red meat and are at risk of iron deficiency anaemia; think about iron deficiency in any consistently pale-looking patient. If this is the case, establishing the cause of the deficiency becomes the next priority when assessing your patient.

Symptoms of iron deficiency

Children	Adults
Blue sclera / rosy cheeks	Hypothyroidism
Fatigue	Loss of concentration
Hyperactivity	Low energy -> irritability
Loss of concentration	Poor immunity/repeated infections.
Low energy -> irritability	Depression
Pallor/dark circles under eyes.	Dysphagia
Pica; chewing paper, dirt, clay, rubber	Fatigue
Poor immunity -> repeated infection	Frequent need to clear throat
Sleep more than 12 hours, waking tired	

Causes of iron deficiency
- Blood loss (bleeding noses, menstruation, haemorrhoids, gastric ulceration, cancer)
- Copper excess (blocks iron uptake)
- Excess dairy products or tea (blocks iron uptake)
- Gut parasites
- Lead or mercury accumulation (blocks iron uptake)
- Low dietary iron
- Malabsorption syndromes

- Medications
- Vitamin C deficiency (Vitamin C enhances absorption of non-haem iron from foods consumed concurrently. Haem iron from animal sources is not affected by vitamin C intake.[15])

A blood test for haemaglobin easily reveals iron deficiency. It is helpful to have ferritin stores tested as well, as the haemaglobin may be normal but ferritin, which measures the body's iron stores, can be low and the patient can still have low energy levels.

A lesser-known consequence of iron deficiency is hypothyroidism. Since 1938[16], it has been understood that iron deficiency can impair thyroid function, by inhibiting the production of the amino acid *tyrosine,* the precursor to *thyroxin.* Therefore it is wise to check the iron status of patients presenting with thyroid disorders.

Treatment
The simplest treatment for iron deficiency anaemia due to dietary lack is to give an iron supplement for the first month or two until the patient (or parent) has an opportunity to fully adjust the diet and while the practitioner has time to consider *the cause behind* the patient's anaemia. In clinic I use *Spatone*[17], which rapidly increases iron levels without causing constipation. To maximise iron absorption, one can also give concurrent doses of *Ferrum Phos 3x.*

These two cases demonstrate how, when thinking only homeopathically, it can be easy to overlook the causation, or 'exciting cause' of your patient's problem.

Examples
Seven year-old boy with bedwetting
This boy had a bedwetting problem that was unresponsive to treatment. He came for his appointment after-school, had huge dark circles under his eye, and was struggling to stay awake. His inner lower eyelids were pale and he looked exhausted without any obvious reason, so he had a blood test, which revealed a low haemaglobin, and an iron supplement was duly given!

At his one month follow up, he had only suffered one or two episodes of bedwetting in the first two weeks after his consultation, and none since. There was no constitutional predisposition to bedwetting – his sleep had been so deep from exhaustion that he was unable to rouse himself to go to the toilet, which the iron supplement corrected.

32 year-old woman with depression
This mother of two young children presented with exhaustion and depression, struggling to get through each day (a common presentation in practice!) She

---

[15] Lynch, S, 'Interaction of Iron with other Nutrients', *Nutrition Review,* 1997; 55(4); 102-110
[16] Watts, D, *Trace Elements and Other Essential Nutrients*: 4th ed, Writer's Block, Texas, 2003 p.112
[17] 100% natural iron food supplement from the mountains of Snowdonia, Northern Wales - available internationally

was diligent with her diet and lifestyle, ate a healthy (mostly vegetarian) diet and did regular yoga. Her mood was improving on antidepressant medication, but her energy levels were still low. After several homeopathic medicines and little response, she was given an iron supplement. After six weeks, her energy had significantly increased and she felt much 'happier.' The change was so profound it leads one to wonder how many women taking anti-depressants are in need of iron supplementation.

Discussion

Why not give Calc Phos, Ferrum Phos or other potentised medicine for nutritional deficiencies?

Experience tells me that these medicines are effective when there is a disorder of iron metabolism but ineffective when there is a frank iron deficiency. The hair mineral analysis below revealed *no tissue stores of iron* in a lethargic young woman who presented with gut problems. Her energy levels did improve with an iron supplement.

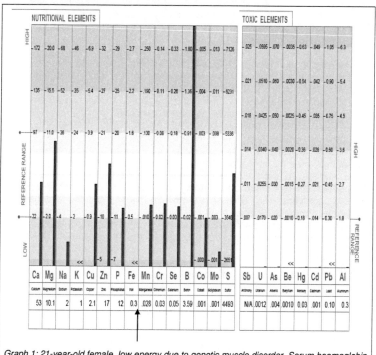

Graph 1: 21-year-old female, low energy due to genetic muscle disorder. Serum haemaglobin normal yet the patient responded well to iron supplementation.

Daily Iron Requirements
Babies and young children: 10-15mg
Teenagers: 18mg
Women: 18mg
Pregnant & lactating women: 25mg
Men: 10mgs

Magnesium

Magnesium Deficiency
Magnesium is the body's natural sedative and is one of the most easily lost minerals when any form of stress occurs. It is a key element for cell metabolism and is involved with hundreds of enzyme systems throughout the body. One of its important roles is to *modify calcium metabolism* within cells and around joints. Magnesium prevents calcium build up in the cells, such as occurs in osteoarthritis, bursitis, and kidney stones. Calcium excess is also found in arteriosclerosis and other cardiovascular disorders such as high cholesterol and blood lipid balance.

Magnesium is also needed for normal sodium and potassium metabolism – too little can lead to sodium excess and therefore, fluid retention. Magnesium deficiency is therefore a crucial element in assessment of hypertension and pre eclampsia. Unfortunately, the main nutritional advice given to most hypertensive patients is to lose weight and 'eat less salt'.

Magnesium and stress
Stress increases the utilisation of magnesium, so prolonged stress may lead to a magnesium deficiency. Levels are also affected by cardiovascular disease, myocardial infarction, toxaemia of pregnancy, hypertension or post surgical complications, excessive vomiting, burns, protein malnutrition, endocrine disorders such as diabetes, parathyroid disease, hyperthyroidism with hypercalcaemia and hyperaldosteronism,[18] which leads to low potassium levels. In naturopathic parlance this is called 'adrenal exhaustion'.

Symptoms of Magnesium Deficiency
- Chronic Fatigue
- Cramps
- Excessive sweating, body odour after little exertion
- Heart disease
- Hyper-irritability, edginess.
- Insomnia
- Jumpiness

---

[18] Groff, J, & Gropper, S, *Advanced Nutrition and Human Metabolism*, 3rd ed, Wadsworth/Thompson Learning, USA, 2000

- Muscle tremors, spasms seizures (epilepsy)
- Osteoporosis
- Paraesthesia (tingling, numbness or other altered sensation)
- Premenstrual Syndrome
- Poor concentration, memory loss
- Pre-eclampsia
- Tremors
- Urinary frequency (bladder muscles unable to fully relax).

Causes of Magnesium Deficiency
- Alcohol excess
- Chemotherapy and other medications, including diuretics
- Chronic bowel disorders/diarrhea and malabsorption syndromes
- Excessive physical exertion
- Heavy metal toxicity; lead, cadmium
- Low intake
- Stress; mental, emotional and physical.

Detecting Magnesium Deficiency
Many deficiency symptoms like cramps and tremors are obvious, and levels are easily checked via a Hair Tissue Mineral Analysis (HTMA). If the magnesium level is lower than the calcium level, a 'relative' deficiency exists. If the level is below the reference range, this is an 'absolute' deficiency. The hair analysis result below indicates that this patient has both an absolute and a relative magnesium deficiency.

When treating homeopathically, it is important to correct the underlying conditions that have caused the magnesium deficiency in the first place. Ongoing stress, gut disorders or other disease can be addressed by homeopathic medicines but to get a prompt, early improvement in patients, a magnesium supplement in conjunction with homeopathic remedies, can be given, and then withdrawn as able. Hair mineral analysis gives an accurate tool with which to monitor magnesium levels.

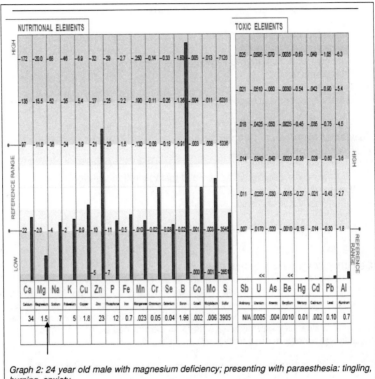

Graph 2: 24 year old male with magnesium deficiency; presenting with paraesthesia: tingling, burning, anxiety

Sometimes, a magnesium deficiency is the sole reason for a patient's presenting symptoms:

Example
24 year-old man with tremors, burning, prickling, tingling and anxiety
This man had had chemotherapy for lymphoma four years previously. He presented with tremors, burning, tingling and anxiety, and was understandably fearful that his malignancy had returned. After just four days taking a magnesium supplement, all his symptoms disappeared. It is well documented that chemotherapy (and other medications) causes magnesium depletion.

Treatment of Magnesium Deficiency
- Correct the diet
- Minimise medications where possible
- Monitor levels through hair mineral analysis
- Normalise gut function
- Supplementation
- Treat existing illnesses.

Low calcium and magnesium levels are common in children with autism spectrum disorders, including hyperactivity, ADD and ADHD. Levels are worth checking, because supplementation can help to calm these children down.

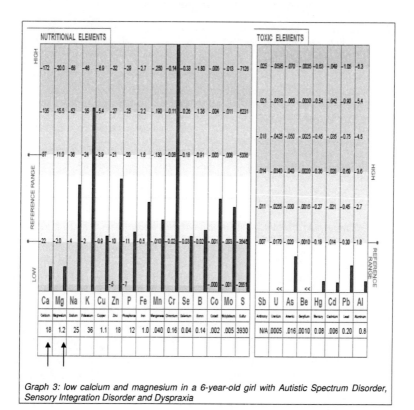

Graph 3: low calcium and magnesium in a 6-year-old girl with Autistic Spectrum Disorder, Sensory Integration Disorder and Dyspraxia

Daily Magnesium Requirements

Infants: 40-70mg
Children: 50-250mg
Adults: 300-400mg
Pregnant & lactating women: 450mg

Zinc

Zinc is a crucial mineral for normal growth and development, immune function, skin health, appetite regulation, endocrine function and immunity. It is essential for the normal function of over 100 body enzymes.

Once you start looking for zinc deficiency, you surely will find it. It is easy to detect – look for white spots on the fingernails. A zinc taste test is also indicative of deficiency and may prove positive even when there are no nail spots present.

It is well known that Australian soils are deficient in zinc.[19] Intensive animal farming and horticulture anywhere in the world challenges zinc levels in soils. When treating patients who constantly get viruses and are unresponsive, or relapse after homeopathic treatment, suspect zinc deficiency. Zinc is specific in killing some viruses on contact.

In chronically ill patients, assessing zinc status is important, because supplementation can bring about rapid improvement of symptoms. In addition to the zinc taste test, Hair Tissue Mineral Analysis (HTMA) is one of the best ways to assess long-term zinc status.

The following two hair tissue mineral analyses show severe absolute zinc deficiency:

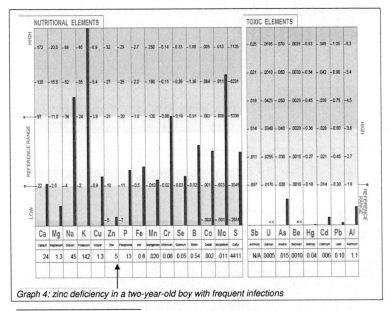

Graph 4: zinc deficiency in a two-year-old boy with frequent infections

---

[19] See for example *www.usyd.edu.au/agric/acpa/people/budi/selenium.htm*

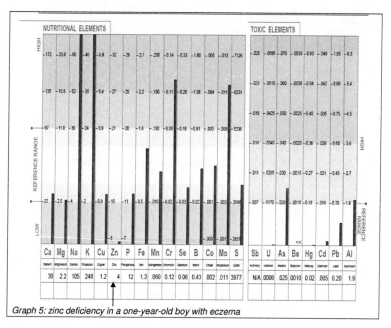

Graph 5: zinc deficiency in a one-year-old boy with eczema

Symptoms (some) of zinc deficiency
- Disturbed sleep
- Loss of smell and taste
- Poor concentration
- Poor wound healing
- Premenstrual Syndrome
- Repeated *viral, yeast and fungal* infections / poor immunity
- Restless limbs
- Stretch marks
- White spots on the fingernails – the most easily recognisable sign.

Diseases associated with zinc deficiency
- Acne and dermatitis
- Autism
- Heavy metal accumulation
- Infertility
- Macular degeneration
- Mental illness; depression, bipolar disorder
- Peptic ulcer
- Prostatic enlargement
- Rheumatoid arthritis
- Skin disease: lupus, scleroderma, psoriasis, yeast and fungal infections.

Causes of zinc deficiency
- Alcohol – high intake
- Copper excess
- Foods grown in zinc deficient soils
- High grain diet (blocks absorption)
- Medications: cortisone, diuretics, anti-depressants, anti- inflammatories
- Poor, or vegetarian diet
- Stress.

Treatment of Zinc Deficiency
Zinc supplementation needs to be monitored because excess zinc can also predispose to *bacterial* infections due to it creating copper deficiency, and this may elevate LDL triglycerides and cholesterol.

Absolute zinc deficiency can be corrected with relatively small amounts of zinc. Monitor tissue zinc accumulation every six months via Hair Tissue Mineral Analysis.

Example

Female, 33: Sinus infections
This woman had repeated non-allergic sinusitis and viral infections, not responsive to antibiotics. She responded well to Silicea but when she stopped taking her zinc supplement, her sinusitis symptoms reappeared. She required prolonged zinc supplementation.

Once you see the extent of zinc deficiency in your patients, and experience the benefits of giving zinc supplements, it is difficult to justify relying solely on homeopathic remedies in some chronic cases. As with other minerals, zinc deficiency is often an obstacle to cure.

Daily Zinc Requirements
Infants – 3-5mg (elemental zinc)
Adults: 15 – 30mg (elemental zinc)

Zinc Absorption
Adequate levels of Vitamin B6 and magnesium are necessary for zinc absorption, and good quality supplements contain these co-factors.

Selenium
Selenium is an important anti oxidant and is vital for normal immune function, as well as an essential tool in auto-chelation of heavy metals. Selenium is important for preventing free radicals from accumulating in human tissue. Unlike iron, magnesium and zinc, the clinical signs of selenium deficiency are not obvious and its deficiency is mainly detected in hair tissue mineral analysis results. Insufficient selenium stores can allow toxic mineral accumulation, particularly mercury and cadmium.

Diseases caused by selenium deficiency
- Auto-immune disorders (eg cancer, cystic fibrosis, Crohn's disease)
- Cardiomyopathy
- Cataracts
- Degenerative conditions
- Haemolytic anaemia
- Heavy metal accumulation
- Thyroid disturbance.

Causes of selenium deficiency
- Alcoholism
- Chemicals
- Drugs
- Heavy metals
- Oxidative stress
- Premature infants
- Selenium deficient soils or poor nutrition.

Nutritional Imbalances

Any vitamin or mineral supplement can cause an iatrogenic disease if taken inappropriately. It is wise then, to be aware of the supplements that your patient is taking and ensure that the supplement is clinically necessary. Mineral levels can easily and safely be monitored via Hair Tissue Mineral Analysis.

This section on nutritional imbalances describes how minerals some relate to one another, and why it is important to understand this when treating some conditions with homeopathy. When minerals are out of balance with each other, specific conditions can develop. The following is far from comprehensive, but is what I have found most often in clinic.

Here, I discuss the relationship between:
- Calcium and magnesium
- Copper and zinc.

Calcium and Magnesium

In a culture where most women, middle aged and older, are taking some form of calcium supplement, practitioners need to be able to assess the impact this has on the patient and how it may affect homeopathic treatment. Calcium supplementation is not *necessarily* needed in every post-menopausal woman and can be an obstacle to cure in itself. The topic of calcium metabolism is vast and discussed only briefly here.

Calcium Deficiency?
Given the abundance of calcium in our food supply, calcium deficiency is one of the *least* likely scenarios to occur in an adult patient. What is more likely is

a calcium *metabolism* problem. Children, particularly those with learning and behavioural disorders, often have low calcium (and magnesium) levels. For proper calcium metabolism, there needs to be equal amounts of calcium and magnesium.

The currently trend for many women to take calcium supplements can be detrimental and it does not address the reason for osteoporosis. A recent report reveals that calcium supplementation can lead to heart disease[20] due to excess calcium build up in body tissue. As stated above, o*steoporosis is seldom a problem of calcium deficiency* in the developed world. More often it is a problem of the relative deficiency of calcium's co-factors, mainly vitamin D, magnesium and phosphorus. If a patient is deficient in magnesium and phosphorus relative to calcium, it can lead to calcium being poorly absorbed into bone tissue and result in osteoporosis. This explains why it is possible to see an osteoporotic patent with calcium excess showing on HTMA. *Calcium status should be assessed on Hair Tissue Mineral Analysis before commencing any supplementation.* In practice, it is more common to see a *young child* with frank calcium deficiency than a post-menopausal woman.

To illustrate the point with osteoporosis, the HTMA below shows that of a woman suffering from severe osteoporosis, yet shows calcium at the highest level of all the minerals. She was prescribed a calcium supplement by her doctor, but this result clearly shows that it was not calcium that she needed.

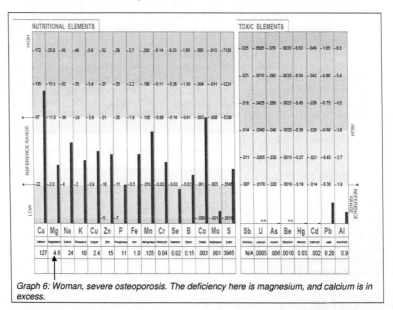

Graph 6: Woman, severe osteoporosis. The deficiency here is magnesium, and calcium is in excess.

---

[20] Research: Effect of calcium supplements on risk of myocardial infarction and cardiovascular events: meta-analysis http://www.bmj.com/cgi/content/full/341/jul29_1/c3691

Other factors affecting calcium levels
- *High* dairy intake (high calcium foods can create a relative magnesium deficiency)
- Vitamin D deficiency (too little sun exposure, oestrogen /insulin deficiency).

Symptoms of Calcium Deficiency
- Anxiety
- Fatigue
- Hyperactiviity (children)
- Hypersensitivity, irritability
- Insomnia
- Muscle cramps
- Palpitations
- Tingling in extremities.

Note how these closely resemble the symptoms of magnesium deficiency.

Causes of Calcium Deficiency
- Antacids
- Cortisone (prolonged use)
- Dairy free diet due to allergy
- Endocrine disorder (thyroid, diabetes)
- High phytate /oxalic acid diet (rhubarb, spinach, beet greens, grains)
- Malabsorption diseases.

Factors Increasing Calcium Demand	Maximising Calcium Absorption
Inactivity (lack of exercise), bed rest	Exercise –one hour 3 times weekly
Lack of sunlight (Vitamin D)	Sensible sun exposure, Cod Liver Oil
High protein diet	Moderate protein intake
Excess sugar, phosphates (soft drinks)	Fresh fruit juices (Vitamin C)
Alcohol, coffee, cigarettes, cortisone,	Minimal drugs and medications
Aluminium (cookware, antacids)	Stainless steel/enamel cookware
Low stomach acid	Lemon juice, apple cider vinegar
Hypothyroidism, diabetes	Hormonal health (thyroid, insulin, oestrogen)
Poor nutrition	Sufficient intake of Vitamins A, C, D, E and magnesium, phosphorous, copper, selenium

Getting proper delivery of calcium into bones is a complex process and requires far more than simple calcium supplementation. Correcting underlying disease (diabetes, kidney, thyroid/parathyroid disease) is important.

Calcium Excess
There is far less emphasis on how many of our patients have too much calcium (hypercalcaemia). Hypercalcaemia predisposes to osteoarthritis. In an effort to excrete the calcium excess, the body deposits its calcium into the

soft tissues. Bony tissue also becomes hypertrophied as the excess calcium is deposited on the periostial tissue as exostoses (bony spurs).

As stated, calcium supplementation, which requires careful monitoring of calcium levels in blood and tissue, should only be prescribed after reference to a Hair Tissue Mineral Analysis (HTMA) and given when really needed.

Symptoms of Calcium Excess (including inappropriate use of Calcium supplements)
- Anxiety
- Depression, crying spells
- Exhaustion
- Fatigue
- Headaches
- Insomnia
- Memory poor, loss of concentration
- Panic attacks.

Women often start taking calcium during menopause, so when treating menopausal women, practitioners need to take this into account.[21] It is a potential iatrogenic obstacle to cure.

Homeopathic treatment
- In post-menopausal women, *Cimicifuga* and *Calcarea Carb* can be given to correct calcium metabolism.
- *Calcarea phos 3x*, twice daily, and *Symphytum 200c,* once every second day, can treat osteoporosis (but check for mineral deficiencies).

Copper and Zinc

By far the main presentation in the copper and zinc relationship (which should be in equal amounts) is an excess of copper relative to zinc. Understanding copper metabolism and balance has been a real breakthrough in my practice and allowed me to succeed in many cases that previously I could not. Copper levels are easy to monitor via hair tissue mineral analysis.

Symptoms of copper excess (toxicity): see Chapter 5 for more detail.
- ADHD[22] mood disorders, poor concentration
- Allergies – respiratory and food
- Anaemia
- Anxiety
- Biliary congestion[23] (copper congests the liver and can occlude the gallbladder and common bile duct)
- Depression
- Poor sleep

---

[21] Watts, D, Ibid
[22] Attention Deficit Hyperactivity Disorder
[23] Biliary congestion is described in:: *The Treatment of Irritable Bowel Syndrome* Gamble, J, *Mastering Homeopathy 2* (2006) p 74

- Premenstrual syndrome (copper rises with oestrogen and is retained in women who use the Pill (OCP) or IUD)
- Restless or fidgety limbs
- Susceptibility to yeast infections.
- Tics and tremors.

Copper Deficiency

While copper excess is more common, deficiency also occurs, with a fascinating list of disorders that can be extremely helpful to practitioners struggling with chronic cases.

Immunity

Copper deficiency predisposes to bacterial infection (zinc deficiency to viruses). Chronic bacterial infections, such as a tooth abscess, can deplete copper stores and cause a vicious cycle of infection and further copper depletion.

Musculo skeletal health

- Copper is crucial to utilise iron properly. Without copper, iron product from normal blood cell breakdown cannot be accessed for new red blood cells. Instead, iron accumulates in joints, creating pain and inflammation. This explains why arthritis patients get pain relief when they wear a copper bracelet. The copper helps to mobilise iron out of the joints. These patients may also present as iron-deficient anaemic, but it is *copper, and not iron* that will bring their haemoglobin back to normal.
- When fighting off a bacterial infection, the body needs copper to fight invading organisms. If this process depletes tissue copper, it is a reason why some patients develop rheumatoid arthritis following a bacterial infection: the low copper stores result in iron saturation of the joints.
- Copper retention occurs naturally during pregnancy, which is why patients who have arthritis suddenly improve when they fall pregnant.
- The musculo-skeletal system needs copper for the normal production of ligaments and spinal discs; some scoliosis patients are copper deficient.

Nervous system

Both copper deficiency and excess have profound nervous system effects and is needed for normal myelination. Patients with multiple sclerosis and Parkinson's disease can show severe copper deficiency on Hair Tissue Mineral Analysis.

Cardiovascular

Atherosclerosis and raised triglycerides can occur when there is a copper deficiency.

Summary of conditions that can be caused by Copper deficiency
- Recurring bacterial infections
- Low density blood lipids (LDL) elevated
- Nervous system disorders such as Multiple Sclerosis
- Rheumatoid arthritis (copper bracelets are popular)
- Skeletal deformities (scoliosis).

Contra indications in copper Deficiency
- Vitamin C supplementation (antagonises copper absorption, so take care; not *all* infections benefit from vitamin C supplementation)
- Zinc supplementation (antagonises copper absorption).

Treatment
- High copper foods (chocolate, brazil nuts) and supplementation, but only if a deficiency has been established on Hair Tissue Mineral Analysis.

Chapter 3
Infection

If a patient is never well since an acute infection such as chicken pox, herpes, glandular fever, it is common practice to give a *nosode*. Similarly, if an acute illness is not responding to the *simillimum*, giving the *nosode* in addition to the *simllimum* is more efficacious.

When the *simillimum* does not reap results, one obstacle can be an underlying or previous infection, which calls for meticulous case taking and demands detailed recall from the patient. Ongoing infection, or the effects of a past infection, is not always obvious.

Hahnemann enunciated the pathogenic basis of chronic diseases when he described the chronic *miasms*. In his day, failure to recognise these *miasms* presented an obstacle to cure; and a *nosode* was needed to advance treatment. The same principle applies when treating patients today who have infections which become chronic.

Streptococcus

Patients who are never well since a severe tonsillitis may have 'hidden' streptococcal infection.

Example
A 9 year old boy had recurring throat infections with classic 'strawberry' tongue, painful swallowing, high fever and leg pain. These infections recurred every few weeks to months, always with similar symptoms. Between episodes he was well, but had less stamina than his two brothers, often complaining of fatigue, poor appetite and vague leg pains. He also had a history of kidney infections as a baby. His chronic picture did not change dramatically until I gave him Streptococcinum in conjunction with Calcarea Phos 200c.

Think of *Streptococcus* when there is a history of 'strep throat' followed by musculoskeletal pain and fatigue. This bacterium can also be responsible for diseases such as nephritis, scarlet fever, necrotising fasciitis, Paediatric Neuropsychiatric Disorder (PANDAS), rheumatic fever and rheumatoid arthritis.[24]

Deep Gum Infection
Patients with deep gum infections can be undiagnosed and may have no signs or symptoms in their gums. Non-specific symptoms are:
*   Blood tests may not necessarily confirm the presence of infection (ESR).
*   fatigue
*   transient fever
*   vague feeling of 'unwellness'.

---

[24] Scammell, H *New Arthritis Breakthrough: the Road Back,* Evans, USA, 1998

Dental X-ray will usually reveal a previously undiagnosed deep gum infection. Failing this, there may be few clues other than the above symptoms, making diagnosis difficult. One possible clue is a history of gum or dental disease: the patient may remark: "I've had trouble with my teeth all my life" and "My headaches are always the same side of my head, and radiate into my ear or jaw."

Example
A 40 year-old man who had suffered from life long fatigue and undiagnosed recurring low fevers with weakness, had assumed it was sequelae from having contracted typhoid. I tried several remedies without any improvement, however some of these caused pain in his teeth. That gave me a clue that gum infection may have been the cause. Further questioning revealed long-standing dental problems. His symptoms were pointing to the problem when prompted by a remedy! It was a bacterial infection that had been underpinning this case for years. Mercurius viv 200c one dose every second day resolved his symptoms.

Mercurius viv 200c has a special affinity for the gum bed.

Post-Viral Syndromes
Three common viruses can produce a picture resembling Chronic Fatigue Syndrome.

Epstein Barr virus and Cytomegalovirus
The sequelae of *Epstein Barr virus* and *Cytomegalovirus* are regularly seen in clinic. Patients report general feelings of fatigue or a vague 'unwell' feeling that lasts for months. If the virus is the only causation and there are no other disease factors present, Chronic Fatigue Syndrome (CFS) of post-viral origin can be treated relatively efficiently.

For post-viral syndromes give:
* The *simillimum* for the presenting symptoms
* *Gelsemium* for fatigue, torpor and cognitive disturbance.
* *Carcinosin* for insomnia, fastidiousness and a family history of malignancy. Include the patient's constitutional remedy when needed.

For cases of 'never well since' Infectious Mononucleosis (Glandular Fever), give the nosode *Coxsackievirus 30c*, which is similar to the triggering virus, one dose every second day for two to four weeks. If this fails, I also use *Cytomegalovirus 30c*, one dose every second day.

Herpes zoster virus
Herpes Zoster (shingles) occurs in people who have had a similar virus, *Varicella* (Chicken pox). *Zoster* can remain dormant in the host's nervous system for years and manifest when conditions are favourable:
* Emotional stress
* Following viral infections
* Deficiency of the anti-viral nutrients zinc and vitamin C.

CFS patients who have *zoster* type symptoms often describe severe muscle pain with a burning, pinching or tingling nature and may also have fibromyalgia. One patient's CFS began after his son contracted Chicken pox. While he did not catch chicken pox, his CFS began a few days after his son was sick, showing a strong susceptibility to the herpes viruses.

If no other remedies are indicated, patients with this type of CFS picture often respond well to *Arsenicum album 200c*, one dose every second day, with intercurrent doses of *Herpes Zoster 1M*. This prescription may need to be given for many months.

Mosquito Born Diseases
Until recently, mosquito-born diseases have not been a primary concern in sub-tropical or temperate climates. Now, the spread of mosquito-born disease is increasing into non-tropical climates, as a likely consequence of global warming. Whichever country you practise in, you are likely to have patients about to travel, who want advice about the treatment of, and protection from mosquito borne diseases:

- Barmah Forrest Virus
- Dengue Fever
- Flavivirus
- Lymphatic Filariasis
- Malaria
- Murray Valley encephalitis
- Rift Valley Fever
- Ross River Virus
- Sindbis Virus Disease
- St. Louis encephalitis
- West Nile Virus – encephalitis
- Yellow Fever.

It is important to know which countries each of these proliferate in and when the high risk seasons are. It is also important to thoroughly inform your patients on mosquito bite prevention measures.

Australia has its share of mosquito borne diseases like Ross River Fever and Dengue Fever. These can cause chronic arthralgia or myalgia and may escape screening because of the absence of more striking symptoms.

When treating *Ross River Virus*, for best results, give the *nosode* of that disease in conjunction with the indicated remedy. For example, in patients with joint and muscle pain in Ross River Fever, prescribe *Rhus tox 30c* with *Ross River Virus Nosode 30c* on alternate days.

Suspect mosquito borne infections when the original symptoms included a fever or vague flu-like symptoms. Careful case taking, especially of the travel history of your non-responding patients, may reveal exposure to a mosquito-borne disease, which will almost certainly require the relevant nosode. Therefore we need to be cognisant of the features of the mosquito borne infections.

Candida (Monilia) Infections

Intestinal candidiasis is a very difficult condition to treat unless one uses the *Candida Nosode* in increasing potencies over many months. Symptoms of intestinal candidiasis are:

- Abdominal bloating
- Fatigue
- Headaches
- Joint pain
- Mood swings
- Oral or genital thrush
- Sinusitis
- Unstable blood sugar

Common Remedies

- Oral thrush: *Borax 30c*
- Genital thrush: *Kreosotum 200c*
- Intestinal candida: *Candida Nosode + Lycopodium 30c* and strict avoidance of sugar.

Treatment of candidiasis has been described in detail elsewhere.[25]

Intestinal parasites

Mastering Homeopathy 2: The Treatment of Irritable Bowel Syndrome, describes the myriad sets of symptoms caused by intestinal parasites, which can be well off the diagnostic radar when evaluating a case. As with other pathogens, when one results in symptoms, a specific remedy needs to be prescribed for that pathogen in conjunction with the *simillimum.*

Eradicating parasites requires a long period of treatment. I find that helminths and amoebic parasites can mostly be treated with *Cina, Stannum Met and Teucrium.* In obstinate cases, I use either the *Trichinose Nosode,* particularly if the parasite is a Helminth. For amoebic infestation, a weekly dose of *Sulphur 200c* in addition to the remedy of choice. The most reliable way to identify intestinal parasites is via a 3-day stool parasitology test.

Significant Medicines For Intestinal Parasites

Listed from the most to the least commonly prescribed.

(a) Cina 200c
(b) Stannum met 200c (+ Nux Vom 30c in some cases)
(c) Teucrium 200c
(d) When residual symptoms persist despite prolonged treatment, next use *Trichinose Nosode,* which should resolve the symptoms.

---

[25] Gamble, J, *Mastering Homeopathy 1*, Karuna Publishing, 2004, p 41. Intestinal candidiasis and dysbiosis is discussed in Gamble, J, *Mastering Homeopathy 2: The Treatment of Irritable Bowel Syndrome*, Karuna Publishing, 2006, p 51

(e) In obstinate cases give *Sulphur 200c*, once weekly. Continue until any aggravation caused by taking the remedy no longer occurs.

Many cases of behavioural problems in children respond well to *Cina,* when they did not respond well to the indicated remedy.

Cina

Cina, the most common remedy used, is described in the *Materia Medicas* with the emphasis on children. However, intestinal parasitosis is equally common among adults and is a major cause of IBS. The irritable child may need *Cina,* however there is another dimension to this medicine. I see patients treated with *Cina* experience improvement in their anxiety. *Anxiety or irritability* are therefore keynotes for prescribing *Cina.* Other symptoms include insomnia, restless leg syndrome, teeth-grinding, rectal and nasal itch, in children *or* adults. Patients requiring Cina have *diarrhoea, more often than constipation*, as part of their IBS symptom picture. My reliable keynote for *Cina* is agitation or irritability of any part of the nervous system.

Each of these medicines is usually given once every second day for at least one month. Key points of *Cina* are:
- Disturbed sleep, including night terrors
- *Emotional disturbance: irritability and/or anxiety*
- Flushes of heat or actual fevers
- IBS symptoms +
  o Itching, prickly heat, or crawling skin sensations
  o Rectal, nasal or palate itching
  o Restless leg syndrome
  o Sinus symptoms in some cases, "allergies"
  o Teeth clenching
  o Vomiting, diarrhoea and constipation.

Stannum Met

In *Stannum,* the irritability and anxiety are not prominent as they are in *Cina.* The focus of symptoms is abdominal pain, around the umbilicus, which the *Materia Medica* for *Stannum* describes. This also is the most common site for parasite-induced abdominal pain. This can be alternated with *Nux vomica,* as discussed below.

Nux vomica

The main complaint is 'never feeling completely empty' after stool. Therefore, patients requiring *Stannum* and *Nux vom* have *constipation more often than diarrhoea. Nux vom* is unnecessary if there is complete bowel evacuation.

Teucrium

Although this is a small medicine in the treatment of intestinal parasitosis, Teucrium has a strong post-nasal symptomatology: with chronic post-nasal drip and/or clinkers, sometimes with nasal polyps. Irritation of the nasal mucosa causes the patient to scratch their nose. Rectal itch is also found with this medicine.

Teucrium also displays no particular mental disturbance. Its other field of action is in adults or children who appear thin and emaciated, no matter how much they eat. Their appetite may be lacking. In these cases, *Teucrium* is more appropriate than *Cina*.

A keynote of *Teucrium* is 'nasal congestion combined with emaciation'.

Trichinose Nosode[26]
This remedy has similar mentals to *Cina* (irritability or anxiety) and can be given when the case keeps relapsing: one d

Mental Illness and Infection

The ability of infection to cause mental disease is gaining increasing attention in medical circles:
- Microbial links are being made to the causes of schizophrenia after exposure to a virus either in utero or early life.
- Mental and behavioural disorders such as Obsessive Compulsive Disorder and neurological symptoms like tics that occur after streptococcal infection (Paediatric Neuropsychiatric Disorder Associated With Streptococcus (PANDAS).[27]

As we know, the tertiary stage of syphilis, caused by the spirochaete *Treponema Pallidum*, causes mental illness. A similar *spirochaete (Borrelia burdorferi)* was identified in the 1970's as the cause of Lyme Disease, the tertiary stage of which also causes profound mental effects. This gives us a new dimension of investigation when assessing patients with mental disturbance: particularly if the cause of the disturbance does not make sense. Now that medical research is revealing a potential link (in *many* studies) between microbes and mental illnesses like schizophrenia, the scope
for our use of potentised organisms, other than the original *miasms*, in clinic takes on new credentials.

The *miasms*:
- Psoric (scabies) *Sarcoptes scabiei.*
- Sycotic (gonorrhoea) *Neisseria gonorrhoeae*
- Syphilitic (syphilis) *Treponema pallidum*
- Tubercular (tuberculosis) organism *Mycobacterium tuberculosis.*

Lyme Disease
There are medically documented cases where patients have been misdiagnosed with mental disease, whereas subsequent testing for and treatment of Lyme disease has resolved their symptoms. As with PANDAS, a bacterium can be responsible for negative emotions and behaviour. In

---

[26] Humans can contract trichiniasis from eating under-cooked meat. It causes diarrhoea and abdominal pain, nausea, periorbital oedema, myalgia, fever, headache. In rare cases there are neurological and pulmonary complications. This nosode is available from selected homeopathic pharmacies.
[27] Insel, Thomas, 'Microbes and Mental Illness'
http://www.nimh.nih.gov/about/director/2010/microbes-and-mental-illness.shtml

homeopathy, where the mental symptoms often take the greatest priority, we must remember the possibility of bacterial infection when our patients, including 'badly behaved' children, do not respond to the well-selected remedy.

Borrelia burgdorferi, the Lyme bacterium, is now widely accepted as a cause of psychiatric disease. The vector for *Borrelia* infection is the deer tick. Long-term sequelae of this infection can cause not only mental or cognitive disturbance, but can easily be confused with Chronic Fatigue Syndrome or fibromyalgia.

Lyme Disease is prevalent throughout the world, especially in Europe and North America, parts of China, Russia and Japan. Yet it is conspicuously absent in Australia – *or is it?* It was discovered in the 1970s after an outbreak of what appeared to be juvenile rheumatoid arthritis in the Old Lyme region of Connecticut, USA.

Lyme Disease has three distinct phases:
1. *Acute:* following the tick bite, a 'bull's eye' type rash appears soon after, or weeks after, the initial bite, called *erythema migrans.* The rash usually lasts for a few weeks. The patient may have forgotten about the bite by the time symptoms appear, making accurate diagnosis difficult, if not impossible. Other symptoms can include vague flu-like symptoms, fatigue and lymph swelling.
2. *Later* – and it may be many years later – the joint inflammatory stage begins. Still the patient will not make any connection between the joint pain and an old tick bite; particularly if he or she has been bitten on many occasions. Some patients develop only vague symptoms of malaise and fatigue, so it is easy to confuse Lyme Disease with Chronic Fatigue Syndrome. Some patients also develop fibromyalgia.
3. *The last stage* centres on the nervous system, affecting cognition, difficulty with concentration, memory loss and distorted or exaggerated sense reception. Paralysis, vertigo or neuralgia may also occur. Meningo-encephalitis, cranial neuritis (especially Bell's palsy) and motor radiculo-neuropathies have also been reported in patients with Lyme Disease.

Common chronic symptoms:
* Fatigue
* Headaches above the eyes
* Poor concentration, "dizzy head". Unable to focus. "Head full of *cotton wool"*
* Recurring 'flus' – aching muscles, heavy head, fever
* Sore joints: knees, wrists, hips, with swelling, redness, heat
* Swollen cervical glands.

Treatment for established or chronic cases of Lyme Disease

Cases with fatigue, malaise, cognitive disturbance
Gelsemium 200c and *Lyme Disease nosode 30c* on alternate days for one month.

Cases with prominent musculoskeletal pain
Rhus tox 30c and *Lyme Disease Nosode 30c* on alternated days.

Prevention
Peter Alex[28] recommends the following protocol for Lyme Disease *prevention*,
Give prophylactically after a tick bite:
Day 1: *Ledum 200c*, one dose
Day 2: *Hypericum 200c*, one dose
Day 3: *Borrelia nosode (Lyme Disease) 30c*, one dose.

Alex goes on to describe *Aurum arsenicosum* as specific for the main Lyme
Disease symptoms. A proving of that remedy is included in his *The
Homeopathic Treatment of Lyme Disease.*[29] In many of the cases presented
by Alex, both *Aurum arsenicosum* and the *Borrelia Nosode* form the central
treatment for established Lyme Disease.

Since less than one in ten cases of Lyme Disease are correctly diagnosed
and documented, consider this possibility in that difficult case consulting you!

Clues that *Borrelia* could be the cause:
• Patient always feels better when taking antibiotics (confirms a hidden
  bacterial infection)
• Patient is never well since a specific disease event (tick bite?)

Summary

The table on the following is not comprehensive, but represents the main
nosodes that I use in practice.

---

[28] Alex, Peter, *The Homeopathic Treatment of Lyme Disease,*HomeopathyWest Publishing, 2006
[29] Ibid

Disease & Organisms Treatment Guide

BACTERIA	Disease	Symptoms
Borrelia burgdorferi (similar to syphilitic spirochaete)	Lyme Disease	Rash, fever, headache, depression, neurological symptoms, arthritis
Streptococcus	PANDAS[30] Paediatric Autoimmune Neuropsychiatric Disorder	Tics, OCD, ADD, ADHD Fixed ideas
Helicobacter pylori	Gastric ulcer	Epigastric pain
Mycoplasma	Pneumonia, Rheumatoid arthritis Autoimmune inflammatory disorders	Unresponsive to usual antibiotic therapy
Staphylococcus	Boils, abscesses, pneumonia,	
PARASITES		
Blastocystis Hominis[31]	'Blastocystis'	Chronic abdominal pain, nausea, bloating, diarrhoea, rectal itch, fatigue
Dientamoeba Fragilis[32]	'Irritable Bowel Syndrome'	**Acute:** Greenish brown diarrhoea **Chronic:** Irritable Bowel, headache, malaise, irritability, weakness
Cyclospora cayetanensis, Giardia lamblia, Cryptosporidium parvum	'Irritable Bowel Syndrome'	Alternating constipation & diarrhoea, abdominal pain, cramping, bloating, flatulence
VIRUSES		
Cytomegalovirus	Silent infection (common) hepatitis, splenomegaly	Fever, miscarriage, stillbirth, pneumonitis
Epstein Barr Virus Herpes Human Virus 4 (HHV4)	Glandular Fever (Infectious Mononucleosis)	Fever, pharyngitis, malaise, lymphadenopathy Chronic Fatigue Syndrome (CFS)
Herpes Simplex Virus (HSV 1, 2 or 3)	Cold sores, genital herpes,	Recurring eruptions, gingivo-stomatitis
Varicella-Zoster	Herpes Zoster, (Shingles) Chicken Pox	Vesicular eruption, nerve pain, post-herpetic neuralgia
YEASTS		
Candida Albicans	Oral, genital, intestinal candidiasis	Itch, discharge, abdominal bloating

Cases exploring the homeopathic treatment of infection are in Chapter 11.

---

[30] http://www.adhd.com.au/PANDAS.htm
[31] http://www.mayoclinic.com/health/blastocystis-hominis/DS00791
[32] http://emedicine.medscape.com/article/997239-overview

Chapter 3: Infection

Chapter 4
Heavy Metal Accumulation

Heavy metals are naturally occurring elements which become toxic if they are accumulated in human tissue. Acute poisonings of toxic elements present clinical pictures that are both medically acknowledged and the subject of provings in homeopathic *materia medicas*: acute effects can be clearly seen. It is patients presenting in my clinic with *chronic* accumulations of toxic elements that have led me to recognising them as obstacles to cure. Chronic accumulations:

- Obstruct a patient's recovery in a homeopathic context
- Produce secondary symptoms in a patient. I emphasise *secondary symptoms*[33] because acute symptoms are fairly homogenous in their presentation, but *secondary symptoms vary greatly from person to person*. Nonetheless, even secondary symptoms of heavy metal accumulation produce a *generic* picture, which can be recognised once one has seen a few patients with the same toxicity. Within this generic picture, the individual particulars appear. Therefore I have identified general 'pictures' which I have found occur clinically in patients suffering from an accumulated burden of one or more toxic elements.

Why is there a strong emphasis on heavy metal toxicity in this book? The reason is that I have found heavy metals to be a common obstacle to cure in practice. Once identified, they can be gently removed with homeopathic medicine. Aggravation is minimal, and improvement is continuous provided the *tautopathic* (homeopathic) remedy is given in conjunction with the *simillimum*. Therapeutic chelation is a controversial, often expensive, process for patients to go through. Using homeopathic medicine to achieve removal of heavy metals, while largely unknown, is comparatively straightforward and inexpensive for the patient.

Homeostasis
First, it is important to understand what heavy metal accumulation is, and to understand its relationship to symptom presentations in our patients.

We live in a biochemical soup, which includes toxic metals. These are just a few examples of the myriad sources of heavy metals:
- Air pollution (cadmium and mercury from coal furnaces)
- Drinking water (aluminium, copper)
- Drinking water may contain naturally occurring toxic elements
- Home (aluminium or copper cookware, pesticides, garden chemicals).
- In vitro accumulation (lead or arsenic from house renovations to prepare the nursery while the mother is pregnant)
- Personal care products eg copper and lead-containing hair dyes

---

[33] Organon, §112-115

- Pesticides still contain arsenic
- Soils used for horticulture may be naturally high in elements such as cadmium and mercury
- Swimming pools (copper)
- Vaccinations (mercury, aluminium).

While there are considered to be 'safe' levels of the toxic elements, the truth is that no level elements like mercury, lead, arsenic, cadmium is 'safe,' as their presence is antagonistic to the nutrient minerals like calcium, magnesium, zinc and selenium.

In health, the body can absorb what it needs from this chemical soup and excrete the rest via the gut and kidneys, which is crucial to maintaining homeostasis. For a variety of reasons, some individuals are unable to adequately excrete toxic minerals, resulting in chronic disease.

Some of these reasons may be:
- Constitutional or genetic propensity (a person who is a 'poor chelator' of a heavy metal may pass that idiosyncrasy to their child. I have seen this in clinic many times, where a parent's toxic metal profile is the same as their children's.)
- Deficiency of the 'protective' minerals, eg zinc protects us from cadmium, mercury and copper.
- Disease event: an acute viral infection can cause retention of copper
- Ongoing exposure, eg dust containing lead, which is common in old houses, or living near a coal-burning plant.
- Poor gut function.

The body's normal process of dealing with a toxic element is to remove it from the bloodstream as efficiently as possible so as to protect the vital organs. If the toxic element cannot be excreted via the organs of elimination, the body will sequester the element of our circulation and deposit it in a safe place: fatty, epithelial or even endocrine tissue. When the toxic load becomes too great after many years of accumulation homeostasis breaks down. It is at this point that symptoms of chronic disease appear.

Measuring Toxic Metals
Hair Mineral Tissue Analysis (HTMA) is a simple tool that we have at our disposal. It is useful in locating long term or past toxic accumulation. These will not be found in blood tests unless they are in large amounts and the exposure is recent (ie an acute exposure or poisoning.) HTMA is discussed in Appendix 2.

Heavy Metal Toxicity
- Acute poisonings with heavy metals produce evident acute symptoms. The *Homeopathic Materia Medica* is rich with vivid descriptions of the proving symptoms of all of the heavy metals like arsenic, mercury, lead, cadmium aluminium and antimony.

- Chronic accumulation of small traces of heavy metals *produces no symptoms at all unless homeostasis breaks down.* It is at this point that the patient seeks treatment.
- While acute poisoning with a toxic element produces *primary* symptom responses in a patient, the symptoms which result from a chronic accumulation produce *secondary* symptoms. Primary and secondary responses are described in Hahnemann's *Organon*, §112-115.

Here are some examples of *different* patient responses to accumulation of the toxic levels of cadmium and copper:

Example
This four year old girl presented with abdominal pain, restless sleep and chronic loose stools. Note the extremely high level of cadmium, mercury and copper accumulation (well off the graph). One would expect her symptoms to be far worse. This patient can tolerate high cadmium toxicity: she has a strong constitution. Nonetheless she has poor ability to excrete the cadmium. Her sister and mother have similarly high cadmium.

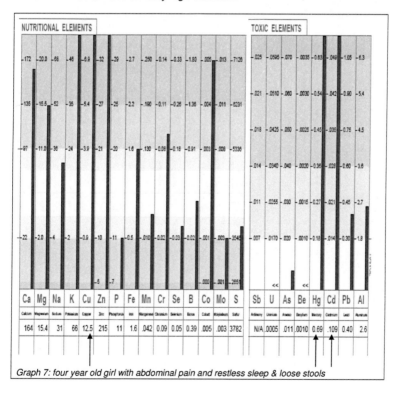

Graph 7: four year old girl with abdominal pain and restless sleep & loose stools

57

Example

This 15-year-old boy presented with Chronic Fatigue Syndrome:

- *Fatigue+++*
- *Nausea+++*
- *Recurring viruses+++*
- *Chronic blocked sinuse.*

He has a similar copper and cadmium load to the patient in the previous example, yet his symptoms were far more severe. Constitutionally speaking, his body is less able to tolerate cadmium (ie his vitality is more greatly affected)

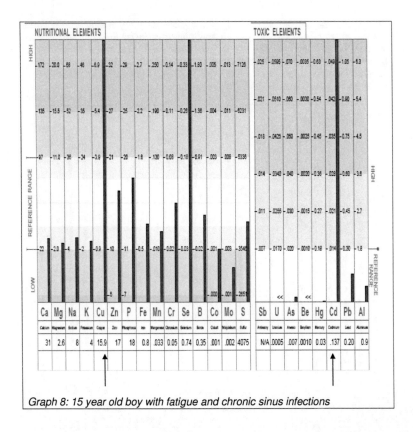

Graph 8: 15 year old boy with fatigue and chronic sinus infections

Chelation

Chelation essentially means 'to bind' and so excrete from the body. A healthy body is able to
- Absorb nutritive minerals
- Chelate or bind toxic metals with sulphur compounds from protein in the diet and remove them via the gut.

An efficient auto-chelation system is needed for good health. A healthy gut and adequate protein intake (sulphur amino acid compounds) are needed to chelate toxic metals (and toxic chemicals). If the body is unable to adequately chelate a metal, it will store it in body tissues. This includes the nutritive minerals as well as the toxic ones, as you will see when I discuss copper. If we cannot adequately chelate minerals, *both mineral deficiency and toxic accumulation can occur.*

Chelation (removal) of heavy metals can be an essential component of treatment of chronic illness. There are several 'medical' ways of removing heavy metals. What is not well known is that homeopathic medicines have this capacity.

Essential Elements for Efficient Chelation

1. Alkaline Environment
Heavy metals are not well chelated in an acidic environment.
- *An alkaline tissue environment* of pH 7.0 or higher is desirable for efficient mineral chelation. Urinary pH (reflective of blood pH) is easily measured during a consultation using a urine dipstick. Saliva/urine test strips are available for patients to monitor their pH
- *Correct mineral balance* is essential for tissue alkalinity. The alkaline-forming minerals *are calcium and magnesium.* Acid-forming minerals are sodium and potassium.
- *Proper protein digestion:* sulphurs derived from protein absorption bind (chelate) metals allowing them to be excreted.
- *Alkalinity of tissues* is achieved by daily fruit and vegetables. A diet high in meat and grains can push the tissues into acidity (below 6.5 pH).

2. Adequate nutrition
Deficiency of nutritive minerals allows the accumulation of toxic elements. Below is a chart of the nutritive minerals that oppose the retention of heavy metals. Sufficient stores of these nutritive minerals are needed for effective natural chelation of their toxic antagonists. In other words, appropriate nutrition and optimum digestive health allows the natural chelation of the heavy metals.

Zinc and selenium are two nutritive elements that protect against heavy metal accumulation. Zinc deficiency, which is alarmingly common, permits the toxic accumulation of cadmium, copper and mercury. (I give a zinc supplement to about 30 per cent of my patients, because they show deficiency on the *Zinc*

Tally[34] taste test or their HTMA.) This is one of many reasons why copper accumulation is the most prevalent type of toxic element accumulation seen in clinic. Copper is discussed in Chapter 5.

Factors preventing chelation
- Individual constitutional (miasmatic considerations) or genetic factors
- Poor gut function – improper secretion of digestive enzymes resulting in poor absorption of nutrients
- Disease events
- Acidic tissue environment (oxidative stress)
- Poor nutrition and mineral deficiency: zinc, selenium deficiency, poor protein absorption
- Chemical exposures resulting in disturbance to normal tissue function.

Mineral Antagonists
Adequate amounts of nutritive minerals are needed to protect against heavy metal accumulation.

Nutritive Mineral	Toxic Antagonist
Selenium	Mercury
Zinc	Mercury; cadmium; copper[35]
Iron	Lead; cadmium
Calcium	Lead

Identifying Heavy Metal Toxicity
I use two methods to determine the presence of heavy metals.

1. TESSOL Test[36]
This instant test of a patient's urine:
- Identifies heavy metal presence in the urine if they are in circulation (ionic)
- It does **not** find metals which are completely sequestered into tissue (ie not in circulation).

2. Hair Tissue Mineral Analysis (HTMA)
HTMA identifies type and amount of toxic elements which have been sequestered out of blood into tissue. Thin of blood as the transit lounge and tissue as the destination. Once the element arrives in tissue it is usually not found in the blood. HTMA is discussed in Appendix 2.

---

[34] *Zinc Tally* is a zinc liquid available for assessing a patient's zinc levels via the subjective mechanism of taste
[35] Although copper is a nutritive mineral, it is also a common toxic mineral when it accumulates in excess. As with any nutritive mineral, too much can cause dysfunction and toxicity.
[36] *TESSOL* is one of many available urine tests used to provide an instant assessment of excretion of heavy metals: see Appendix 1

Treating Heavy Metal Toxicity

Natural Chelation Methods

The longer heavy metals have been resident in human tissue, the more difficult to remove them. This is particularly true for lead and aluminium which, when accumulated over many years, can be sequestered into bone tissue, which may then take years to remove. One case of chronic fatigue and neuritis, caused by chronic lead accumulation, had achieved only minimal improvement despite years of various different chelation methods. These very obstinate cases have 'deeply sequestered' heavy metals, and are discussed at the end of this chapter.

Proprietary supplements are available to gently chelate heavy metals. They are slow in action, so side effects are unusual.[37]

- Marine algae (*Spirulina, Algotene* etc)
- Vitamin C (effective, with zinc, for reducing high copper, but should not be taken if copper is low)
- *Zeolite* – good reputation for chelating aluminium and lead
- *Footsies* – good for children, apply them to the soles at bedtime
- *CH77*: an oral chelation liquid containing low potency alkalising minerals[38]
- *Homeopathic chelation* is what I more frequently use, especially indicated where there is a *specific metal* present, and that metal is causing the presenting symptoms.

Homeopathic Chelation

Homeopathic chelation is useful when:
1. Symptoms are clearly caused by a single heavy metal
2. Symptoms are *maintained by the presence of a heavy metal and may be unresponsive to normal homeopathic treatment.* In other words, the metal forms an obstacle to cure by blocking the therapeutic benefit of a well-indicated remedy. (Mercury has a reputation for doing this.)

In cases where one heavy metal is identified as either causing an obstacle to cure, or is producing the disease symptoms, I use that heavy metal, given *therapeutically* in a mixed potency: 6c/12c/30c/200c and call it a homeopathic 'Chelate'

For example, to chelate mercury I prescribe "*Mercury Chelate*" containing *Mercurius Sol 6c, 12c, 30c, 200c,* together in one bottle, and prescribe it once every second day for at least one month. Obviously, the posology varies, depending on:
- Sensitivity of the patient
- Amount of mercury accumulation shown on the HTMA
- Speed of improvement in the symptoms.

---

[37] See Appendix 1 for a list of these proprietary products
[38] www.harmonology.com.au

Some cases need the *Mercury chelate* (or respective chelation remedy) for many months. A general rule of thumb is to decrease the frequency of dose by one day each successive month, provided that improvement is continuing. For example, in month 2, give *Mercury Chelate* once every *third* day. For each of the four toxic elements, including copper, give this chelation formula. If a nutritive mineral, such as zinc or selenium is deficient on HTMA, the patient needs a supplement as well. Most importantly, I give the similimum on the alternate days between the metal chelate.

Effective Chelation of Heavy Metals with Homeopathy + Mineral Antagonists

Toxic Element	Chelation formula	+ Mineral antagonist
Cadmium	Cadmium Chelate (Cad met 6c, 12c, 30c, 200c)	Iron, zinc
Copper	Copper chelate (Cup met 6 c, 12c, 30c, 200c	Zinc, Vitamin C, iron
Lead	Lead chelate (Plumb met 6c, 12c, 30c, 200c)	Calcium
Mercury	Mercury chelate (Merc sol 6c, 12c, 30c, 200c)	Zinc, selenium

In the next chapter I discuss in detail how to use these homeopathic chelations protocols with the four toxic elements commonly seen in practice. Also see the case examples in Chapter 9.

The *Simillimum*

The *Simillimum* remains the gold standard of homeopathic prescribing. Like any homeopath, I have seen the *similimum* alone cure chronically ill patients with heavy metal toxicity. But what if the patient is a 'non responder'? Few would dispute that the *simillimum* does not achieve cure in all patients. Out of absolute necessity, I have, over the years developed this chelation method and seen greatly enhanced results when the case has been 'stuck' for months or years. Giving the *simillimum* in conjunction with the homeopathic chelation formula has been an exciting development in my practice.

Homeopathic Chelation Method Summary

- *Simillimum:* once, twice or three times weekly (guided by the patient response)
- *Homeopathic chelation remedy:* once every second day, on the alternate or different day to the *simillimum*.

Very Obstinate Cases: Deep Sequestration of 'Hidden' Heavy Metals

In deep sequestration, the body deposits toxic metals so efficiently that they are not excreted at all – not even in the hair, which can be the case in autistic spectrum disorders. Mercury in particular may not be seen on the first HTMA but will appear on subsequent HTMA's after six or twelve months of *simillimum* and chelation therapy. It is a positive sign when toxic elements start to appear on HTMA, even if it results in more symptoms developing.

Example

This 32 year-old man with a malignant brain tumour (astrocytoma) needed oral chelation therapy using CH77[39], one of the general chelation agents, for 12 months before we could see what his toxic load looked like. He also had a selenium supplement. His two HTMA's were taken before and after this chelation therapy. Graph 9 shows his status prior to chelation:

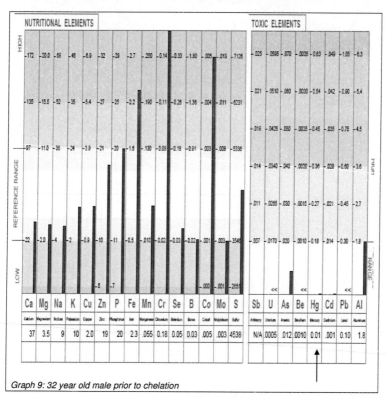

Graph 9: 32 year old male prior to chelation

---

[39] CH77 is an oral chelation liquid containing low potency alkalising minerals

The same man, after 12 months of general chelation, reveals deeply sequestered layers of aluminium, arsenic and mercury (see below). I gave him 12 months of general chelation with CH77[40] and selenium. His urinalysis (TESSOL[41]) continuously showed a strong heavy metal presence during this time. The graph below shows what this treatment had removed from his tissue: note the sudden appearance of mercury in the sample.

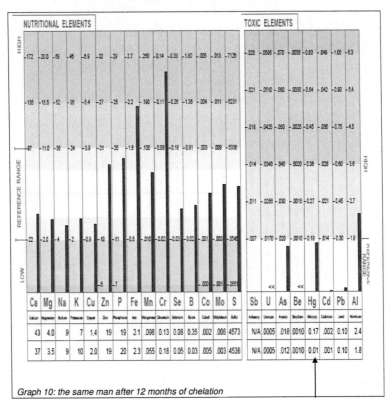

Graph 10: the same man after 12 months of chelation

---

[40] CH77 is an oral chelation liquid containing low potency alkalizing minerals
[41] TESSOL is an instant heavy metal test kit which can be used to test patients' urine

Example

*This woman (below) with chronic migraines, depression and insomnia, had a toxic load of copper. Initial treatment reduced her copper from 31.7mg% to 17.4mg%. After a course of Copper Chelate, one dose every second day, she began excreting more copper: the number **increased** again to 23.9mg%. In other words the specific targeting of her copper revealed a deeper seam of that element, which was excavated by taking Copper chelate. When the body is unable to maintain efficient homeostasis, it must sequester a toxic element into tissue to protect the viability of the vital organs.*

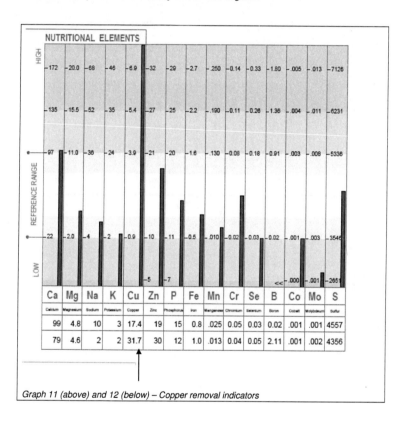

Graph 11 (above) and 12 (below) – Copper removal indicators

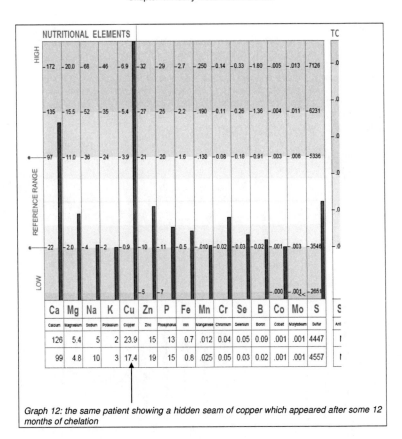

Graph 12: the same patient showing a hidden seam of copper which appeared after some 12 months of chelation

Chapter 5
Common Heavy Metals

Chronic accumulation of heavy metals is a common finding in clinic. When we have patients with Chronic Fatigue Syndrome, neurological disease or unexplained fatigue, and well-selected remedies have not worked, think about heavy metals. When the patient improves and repeatedly relapses, we need to find a sustaining cause. This chapter discusses how that sustaining cause, in the form of heavy metals, can be addressed with homeopathy.

We are all regularly exposed to small traces of elements. A healthy body can adequately chelate (excrete) these traces. Exposure to a large dose of a toxic metal can also occur. This may produce immediate, acute symptoms or there may be a sudden "illness" which appears shortly after the exposure. While acute symptoms are evident, slow accumulation of small amounts is insidious and difficult to detect. Ongoing exposure to a toxic element which is not able to be excreted can give rise to chronic disease and may form an obstacle to cure.

The best method of detecting chronic accumulation is Hair Tissue Mineral Analysis (HTMA).

This Chapter discusses chronic accumulation of four elements which create definite symptom pictures and are commonly seen in clinic. There are other toxic elements which are assayed in Hair Tissue Mineral Analysis, such as arsenic, antimony, uranium, beryllium and aluminium. However, I have not yet seen any clear clinical pictures associated with these toxic elements. Chronic accumulation elicits what Hahnemann described as a *secondary response;* that is, the patient's individual response once the toxicology of the element has been absorbed. Acute poisonings, which are not discussed here, elicit a primary symptom response, the clinical pictures of which are well documented and different to the clinical pictures which occur in chronic accumulation.

I have chosen four toxic elements which I commonly find in practice. Excreting these from the patient's tissue results in a restoration to health. Three of these are heavy metals, viz, cadmium, lead and mercury, which can have a toxic effect even in small amounts; any amount in human tissue is too much. The other of these is the nutritive element, copper, which exerts a significant effect on human tissue when in excess. Excess copper is the most common toxic accumulation that I see in patients.

While they appear from time to time, I have not found the other heavy metals occur commonly in my practice.

Cadmium

Clinical Snapshot of a Patient with Chronic Cadmium Accumulation
Fatigue is the keynote, with trouble waking in the morning. Once awake, it takes a long time to get going into the day. The patient catches every cold and flu which is about. Sometimes there are headaches. Concentration is difficult, not because of restlessness but the head feels heavy and it is a challenge to focus for long. Because of the unrefreshing sleep, the patient has been diagnosed with Chronic Fatigue Syndrome.

Cadmium has earned its toxic reputation largely from industrial emissions. Burning fossil fuels, smelting, metal refining and the use of solder, are all sources. In agriculture, soils and some phosphate fertilisers contain cadmium.

When a cadmium particle, as with all of the heavy metals, enters the air, it binds to smaller particles. It falls to the ground or into the water in rain or snow, and may contaminate fish, plants and animals. Improper waste disposal and spills at hazardous waste sites may cause cadmium to leak into nearby water and soil. The following exposures to cadmium can cause serious health problems:

- Breathing air that contains high levels of cadmium
- Eating food containing relatively high levels of cadmium (eg, shellfish, liver, kidney meats—but the highest levels are often found in potatoes and leafy vegetables)
- Drinking water contaminated with cadmium
- Breathing in cigarette smoke: smoking doubles the average daily intake of cadmium.[42]

A graphic picture of cadmium toxicity was seen in Japan, where cadmium-laden rice was consumed by a large community, with subsequent development of symptoms called 'Itai-Itai' disease.[43] In chronic, toxic accumulations of cadmium, osteoporosis, osteomalacia and kidney disease are well documented.

Our food also contains cadmium, as some soils are high in naturally occurring cadmium.[44] There is an area in New South Wales, Australia, between the towns of Kiama and Nowra, where a large number of patients have high tissue cadmium. Whether this is from the soil, or the proximity to the coal burning industries of Port Kembla in the north, and the paper manufacturing plant at Nowra in the south, has not yet been determined.

However, I see cadmium in patients long before cadmium toxicity is evident in their blood tests: chronic accumulation can start producing subtle symptoms

---

[42] University of Pittsburgh Medical Centre:
http://www.upmc.com/healthatoz/pages/healthlibrary.aspx?chunkiid=120796
[43] http://www.kanazawa-med.ac.jp/~pubhealt/cadmium2/itaiitai-e/itai01.html
[44] Managing Cadmium in Vegetables
http://www.dpi.nsw.gov.au/agriculture/horticulture/vegetables/soil/cadmium

of long before this. The amounts are evident in the Hair Tissue Mineral Analysis (HTMA)

Sources of Cadmium
- Burning plastics
- Coal fired industry
- Electronics industry
- Galvanised water pipes
- Mining, smelting and refining
- Nickel-cadmium domestic batteries
- Paper mills
- Soil and the foods grown in it
- Superphosphate fertilisers
- Tobacco
- Zinc smelters.

Exposure
- City living
- Diet
- Heavy industry – see above.

Toxic Effects of Chronic Cadmium Accumulation
- Anaemia
- Anosmia
- Carcinogen (lung and prostate)
- Fatigue+++
- Insomnia or unrefreshing sleep
- Kidney disease
- Learning difficulties in children (see also lead)
- Vague, recurring flu-like symptoms.

Provings
The Provings of *Cadmium* elicit these general symptoms:
- Extreme prostration with nausea
- Icy coldness during fever
- Worse after sleep (= unrefreshing sleep).

Cadmium is therefore a principle cause of, and remedy for, Chronic Fatigue Syndrome, whose keynote is unrefreshing sleep.

Removing Cadmium
- Zinc (antagonist): 1 tablet daily of approximately 30 mg of elemental zinc, if there is an absolute zinc deficiency (below the reference range) Check for zinc deficiency in relation to copper, cadmium and mercury. Relative deficiency requires higher levels of zinc supplementation. With any ongoing supplementation, HTMA's should be checked every 3-6 months to monitor levels.

- *Cadmium chelate*: one dose every second day, as discussed (one bottle containing homeopathic potency chords of *Cadmium met* 6c, 12c, 30c, 200c). Give in alternation with the *simillimum*.

Note: If cadmium is removed too rapidly it will produce vague flu-like symptoms.

Example
This 13 year-old boy had insomnia and unrefreshing sleep. The insomnia comes from his high copper, while the unrefreshing sleep is more a consequence of the cadmium accumulation.

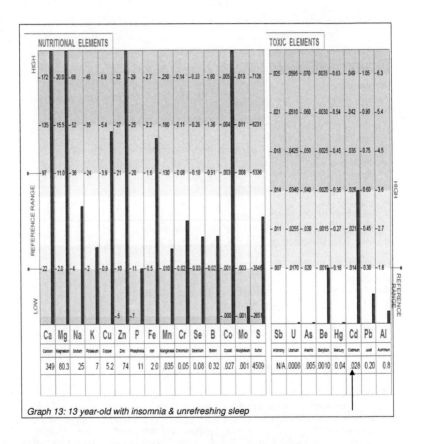

Graph 13: 13 year-old with insomnia & unrefreshing sleep

Example

This young teenage girl had fatigue, learning difficulties (despite being very intelligent), skin infections. This is Case 1, which is discussed in Chapter 9.

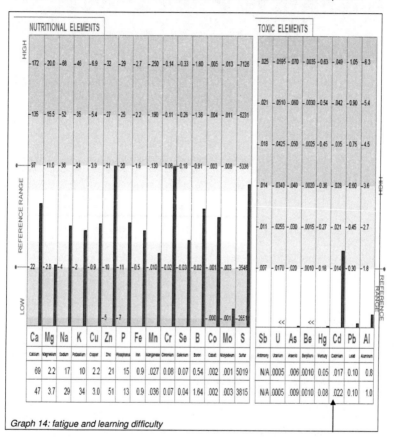

Graph 14: fatigue and learning difficulty

In another case a 70 year old man presented with early (undiagnosed) kidney disease. He had constant pain in his loin, worse early morning, with fatigue. Despite the orthodox view that there is no recovery from cadmium-induced kidney disease, this man fully recovered, with normal kidney function, after six months of treatment with: *Berberis 200c*: one dose every second day; and on each alternate day, *Cadmium Chelate*, one dose.

Copper

Clinical Picture of a Patient with Chronic High Copper Accumulation

The copper child is hyperactive. His limbs are always fidgety. He may have temper tantrums. It takes him over an hour to fall asleep. In the classroom, he cannot concentrate. He complains of headaches, sometimes abdominal pain. He has tics – of the face, neck or hands. Many high copper children will have a diagnosis of ADHD or Asperger's Syndrome.

The copper woman has recurring thrush. She has painful menses, when headaches are worse. She has a tendency to depression that is worse at ovulation and menses. Ever since using the Oral Contraceptive Pill, she has had abdominal bloating, with lots of wind, alternating constipation and diarrhoea. She has food allergies, which trigger headaches and Irritable Bowel Syndrome.

The copper man may have obsessive compulsive tendencies, sometimes with rage. He has insomnia, restlessness, tics and headaches. He has recurring viral infections – he catches every cold that is going around. He has poor concentration. He has skin and respiratory allergies to both airborne and ingested allergens.

Although copper is classed as a nutrient mineral, in excess it causes disease symptoms.[45] This is potentially true for any mineral, however copper excess is the most common elemental toxicity in clinic, and underpins many cases of ADHD and neurological disturbance, especially in young people.

While copper is contained in many foods, those foods are not the cause of copper accumulation in patients affected with copper toxicity. Excess copper is likely to be a combination of exogenous exposure, zinc deficiency and/or genetic predisposition. Despite the source and cause, I recommend that patients with excess copper should reduce the amount of copper containing food sources in order to avoid potential symptom aggravations.

The reasons for excess copper accumulation are vast. Here are some important points:

Xenoestrogens cause Copper Accumulation

Xenoestrogens are industrial or pharmaceutical compounds which exert an oestrogenic effect in human tissue. As with naturally-occurring oestrogen, an excess of xenoestrogens causes retention of copper.[46] Some examples of xenoestrogens are:

- Erythrosine (FD & C Red No 3).
- Parabens (lotions)
- Perfluorinated compounds (PFCs) – the now banned flame retardants.

---

[45] Bremner, I, 'Manifestations of Copper Excess' *American Journal of Clinical Nutrition,* Vol 67, 1069S-1073S

[46] Watts, D, *Trace Elements and other Essential Nutrients,* Writer's BLOK, USA, 2003, p 86

- Pesticides (*DDT, DDE, Dieldrin, Ensosulfan, Lindane, Chlordane*), including common household products – eg fly spray
- Phenosulfathiozine (red dye)
- Pthalates (in plastic food containers, lunch wrap and plastic water bottles; all plastic items numbered 3 or 7on their base.

Further discussion of xenoestrogens can be found in Chapter 6.

Zinc Deficiency

Zinc deficiency allows copper to accumulate in tissue. Since they are antagonists, copper excess depletes zinc stores. I estimate that I give a zinc supplement to about a third of my patients, because their zinc levels are low in the *Zinc Tally* taste test (see Appendix 1) or on their Hair Tissue Mineral Analysis (an orientation of HTMA is in Appendix 2). Zinc deficiency is a common reason why copper accumulation is the most prevalent type of toxic mineral found in clinic. Copper occurs naturally in many foods and is likely to be found in many public water systems. For this reason, and the negative effects of environmental xenoestrogens, discussed in Chapter 6, it becomes clear why high levels of copper have become a health issue.

Sources of Copper other than food

- Hormones (Oral Contraceptive Pill, Hormone Replacement Therapy), Copper Intra Uterine Device.
- Chlorinated swimming pools – a copper compound is the fungicide
- Genetic predisposition
- Drinking water (copper pipes in the house or en route to the house)
- Environmental xenoestrogens
- Vitamin tablets: many supplements contain Copper Amino Acid Chelate, used for copper deficiency, but deficiency is less common than copper excess. Make sure your high copper patients are not taking a supplement containing copper!

High Copper Foods

Almond	Lobster
Avocado	Mushroom
Baker's yeast	Peanut butter
Bran flakes	Pecan
Brazil nut	Shrimp
Chocolate	Sesame seed
Crab	Sunflower seed
Grape	Trout
Haddock	Walnut
Herring	
Liver	

These foods contain microscopic amounts of copper. Environmental and iatrogenic sources are the relevant factors in copper accumulation, not foods. A child born to a parent (male or female) who has high copper may commence life with an inherited high copper burden. I have seen this many times when comparing HTMA results between family members.

Toxic effects of Chronic High Copper Accumulation

A graphic picture of acute copper toxicity is seen in Wilson's disease, a genetic condition which results in the accumulation of copper and liver damage. Neurological symptoms like dyspraxia are also common in this disease.[47]

Neurological
- Hyperactivity
- Headaches and migraines
- Restless limbs
- Restless sleep including insomnia
- Tics.

Cognitive/Psychological
- Poor emotional control; easy frustration and temper tantrums
- Poor concentration (including ADD and ADHD)
- Obsessive Compulsive tendencies.

Pathogenic susceptibility
- Fungal infections – tinea; pityriasis, etc
- Intestinal parasites – helminths, amoebas, etc
- Viruses – especially Epstein Barr; cytomegalovirus, etc
- Yeast infections – monilia (candida albicans.)

Allergic sensitivity
- Airborne allergens – pollens, etc
- Food sensitivities – especially high copper foods and salicylates (migraine after eating chocolate – suspect high copper!).

Biliary system:[48]
- Aggravation from oily, fatty or spicy foods
- Biliary and gallbladder 'sludge'
- Diarrhoea or constipation
- Flatulence, abdominal pain
- Gallstones
- Nausea
- Pale stools.

Mood
- Anxiety
- Depression and insomnia
- Withdrawal

---

[47] Kitzberger, R, et al, 'Wilson Disease', *Metabolic Brain Disease* 2005, Dec; 20(4), 295-302
[48] Category 7 Biliary Stasis: Gamble, J *Mastering Homeopathy 2: The Treatment of Irritable Bowel Syndrome,* Karuna Publishing, 2006, p 74

Hormonal
- Premenstrual syndrome with headaches, constipation, depression, fatigue, weight gain, bloating. (Copper effects increase when oestrogen rises. Patients with oestrogen dominance[49] usually have excess copper.)

Provings

The *Provings* of *Cuprum Met* (Copper), showing an affinity for the nervous system, elicit these general symptoms:
- Chorea
- Coldness with hypoxia
- Dizziness
- Nausea
- Spasms, contractures, convulsions, cramping, tonic and clonic.

Removing Copper

- Zinc (antagonist)[50] – 1 tablet daily of approximately 30 mg of elemental zinc, if there is an absolute zinc deficiency (below the reference range) Check for zinc deficiency in relation to copper, cadmium and mercury. Relative deficiency requires higher levels of zinc supplementation. With any ongoing supplementation, HTMA's should be checked every 3-6 months to monitor levels. Vitamin C will help to antagonise copper retention. In adults give 1000 mg daily.
- Hepatic support, such as *Chelidonium*, since copper congests the biliary system. *Chelidonium* herbal extract 1:2 strength: 10 to 20 drops in water 3x daily. High copper patients who have digestive disease will usually benefit from this treatment concurrent with chelation therapy.
- *Copper chelate*: one dose every second day (one bottle containing homeopathic potency chords of *Cuprum met* 6c, 12c, 30c, 200c). This may be given in alternation with the *simillimum.*

---

[49] Gamble, J, *Mastering Homeopathy: Accurate Daily Prescribing for a Successful Practice*, Karuna Publishing, 2004, p 45
[50] Gaetke, L, et al, Copper Toxicity, Oxidative Stress and Antioxidant Nutrients, *Toxicology,* 2003 doi:10.1016/j.physletb.2003.10.071

Example

This 20 year-old male had food sensitivities with allergic symptoms bordering on anaphylaxis: hives, difficulty breathing. He also experienced anxiety. His copper level is more than two times off the graph. This is Case 2, which is discussed in Chapter 9.

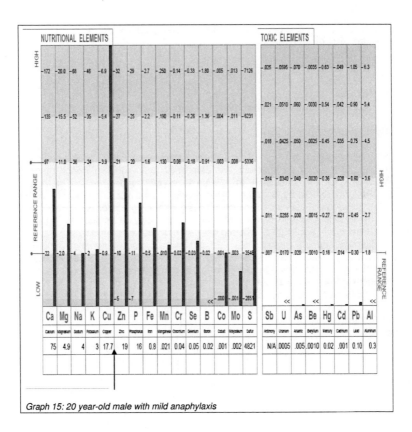

Graph 15: 20 year-old male with mild anaphylaxis

Example

This nine year-old boy was diagnosed with Asperger's syndrome and ADHD. His copper is almost four times off the graph. See Case 6 in Chapter 9.

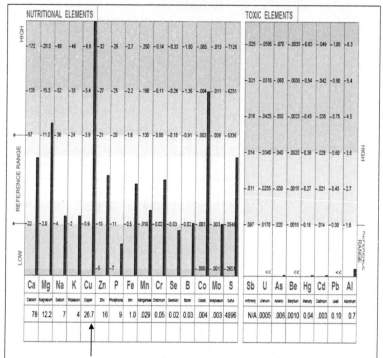

Graph 16: Prescribing both the *similllimum and Copper chelate, his symptom improvement is parallel with the decrease in cellular copper accumulation, as his second HTMA eight months later shows (Graph 17).*

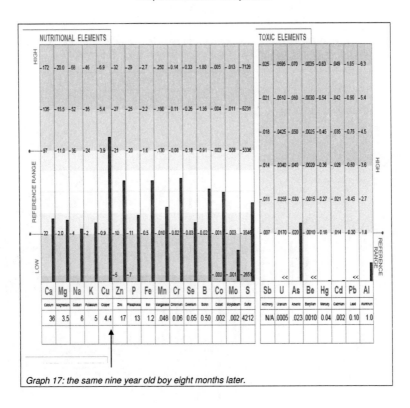

Graph 17: the same nine year old boy eight months later.

Lead

Clinical Picture of a Patient with Chronic Lead Accumulation
He has fatigue, headaches. There is a deep foggy feeling inside the head which creates a feeling of depersonalisation. Diffuse muscle pain has been diagnosed as fibromyalgia. Memory is difficult, even for significant life events. There is deep bone pain which has been diagnosed as arthritis. He has noticed a progressive loss of strength in the muscles – sometimes there is paresthesia (tingling). He has obstinate constipation with abdominal pain. Children have learning difficulty, fatigue and developmental delay in addition to the symptoms described for adults.

As humans have been using lead for thousands of years, history is rich with vivid descriptions of lead poisoning:

- Painter's colic (from ingesting lead based paint), was a common phenomenon: was Caravaggio's violent nature, as seen in his famous paintings, a result of lead poisoning?
- The use of lead utensils and cosmetics is thought to have accelerated the decline of the Roman Empire.

No safe amount of lead exposure has been determined, which means even small traces can produce profound effects. Today there is much lead in both soil and dust in old buildings which has accumulated from decades of using leaded petrol.[51]

Children are possibly most at risk, particularly from lead found in dust and soil from deteriorating (or removal of) lead-based paint in old houses[52]. Children with toxic accumulation may refuse to play or display hyperkinetic or aggressive behaviour disorders.[53]

It is the central nervous system which is most at risk from lead; thus medical literature is full of neurological symptoms: difficult concentration (a 'leaden' head), tremor and muscle weakness, cognitive defects and headaches. Poor appetite, abdominal pain, memory loss, depression and anaemia are also well known symptoms of lead poisoning.

Sources

As with the other toxic elements, in clinic we can see clear pictures of lead accumulation long before lead is seen in blood tests. It will be evident in Hair Tissue Mineral Analyses and can produce the types of symptoms described below.

---

[51] Rossi, E (1 May 2008). "Low level environmental lead exposure - a continuing challenge" (Free full text). The Clinical Biochemist. Reviews / Australian Association of Clinical Biochemists **29** (2): 63–70. ISSN 0159-8090
[52] Pearce, J. M. S. (2007). "Burton's line in lead poisoning". European neurology **57** (2): 118–119.
[53] Pearce, ibid

- Certain heavy industries, eg electroplating, smelters
- Glazes on ceramics
- Lead crystal
- Lead pipes
- Leaded paint in old houses
- Leaded petroleum
- Occupational (scrap metal; glass-makers, etc)
- Some cosmetics, lipsticks and hair colourings.

Toxic Effects of Lead Accumulation
- Abdominal pain
- Constipation
- Deep bone pain (after many years accumulation and can be misdiagnosed as osteo-arthritis)
- Does lead cause brain tumours? – see the examples below
- Fatigue
- Fibromyalgia (also with aluminium)
- Headache
- Hypersomnolence or difficulty falling asleep
- Immune system suppression
- Iron deficiency anaemia
- Muscle weakness / peripheral neuropathy (wrist or foot drop are classical signs of lead toxicity)
- Poor memory.

Children
Delayed development or learning
Hyperactivity or lethargy
Same symptoms as for adults
Unexplained irritability or aggression.

Provings
The *Provings* of *Plumbum Met* (Lead) also show strong neurological symptoms:
- Blue gum line
- Constipation
- Constrictive abdominal colic
- Depression
- Muscle paralysis
- Muscular atrophy
- Tinnitus.

Removing Lead
- If the patient is low in tissue calcium, a calcium supplement may assist the removal of lead, particularly if the lead lies in bony tissue. In these cases, one wants the calcium to be absorbed into the bony tissue as the chelation treatment slowly starts to extract the lead. Be sure the patient has the co-

factors required for correct calcium absorption: adequate digestion; vitamin D, magnesium and phosphorus.

- *Plumbum chelate* (one bottle containing homeopathic potency chords of *Plumbum met* 6c, 12c, 30c, 200c): one dose every second day. This may be given in alternation with the *simillimum*.
- Give iron supplement if low in iron (iron is also an antagonist).

Example

This patient, a six year old girl, has an astrocytoma. Her amount of lead accumulation is twice off the graph. As with the earlier patient with an astrocytoma, there is also a significant presence of mercury.

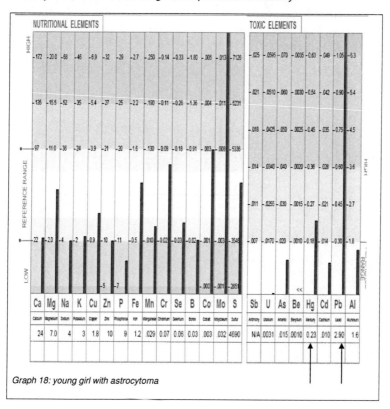

Graph 18: young girl with astrocytoma

Example

A 40 year old woman had chronic headaches, fatigue, fibromyalgia and irritable bowel syndrome, all of which were cleared once her lead load was removed.

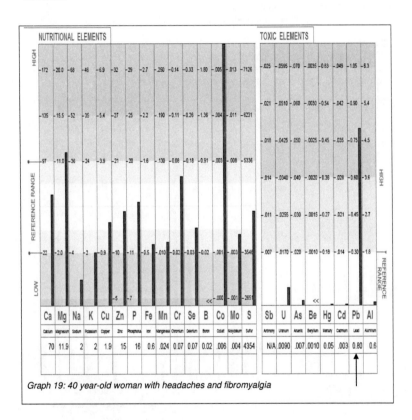

Graph 19: 40 year-old woman with headaches and fibromyalgia

82

Example

A 38 year old woman had fatigue, insomnia, 'inability to think clearly', with a previous history of severe Chronic Fatigue Syndrome. Note that the lead reading is 10 times off the graph. Despite effective homeopathic treatment, her foggy head did not clear up until I gave her homeopathic lead chelate. See Case 3 in Chapter 9.

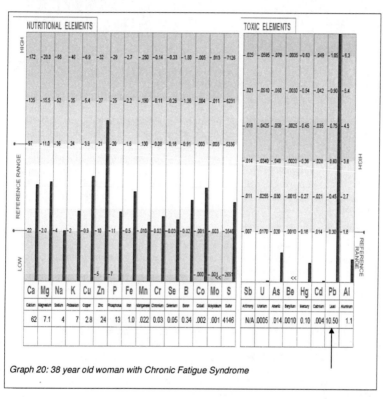

Graph 20: 38 year old woman with Chronic Fatigue Syndrome

Mercury

Clinical Picture of a Patient with Chronic Mercury Accumulation
The patient is oversensitive to all medicines, including homeopathic remedies and may experience an aggravation without improvement of symptoms. There is significant gut disturbance, with abdominal pain, diarrhoea, colitis, and often an intestinal permeability issue ('leaky gut), with disturbances in concentration, mood, energy and cognition after eating certain foods. As with copper, mercury provides a favourable environment for intestinal parasites. There is anxiety, a foggy head, thyroid disturbance, ulceration of mucous membranes and dermatitis. Patients have unexplained fatigue which is usually associated with a 'foggy head'. Autistic children are likely to have deeply sequestered (hidden) mercury.[54]

The only metal which is liquid at room temperature, mercury is still used widely. The light which comes on automatically when you open the car door or your refrigerator has a tilt switch containing mercury, as did the silent light switches popular in the 1970s (now we have mercury-free ones which go 'click'). Unfortunately, in our efforts to reduce energy consumption and carbon emissions, we have placed long life light globes in our homes which contain mercury gas. Emissions from coal burning plants contain mercury the locations of which are linked with the incidence of autism.[55]

Mercury in our silver tooth amalgams has been discontinued in some countries. Some patients are particularly sensitive to the degradation of their mercury amalgams and have to have them replaced. Mercury was placed in amalgams not only because of its versatile pliability, but because it is antiseptic and antifungal – in other words it gets rid of potential dental infections.

Dietary mercury is another common route into human tissue, largely found in seafood, especially the larger fish. It is no surprise then that mercury toxicity is high in many Japanese people, whose main diet is seafood. In 1956 a famous poisoning of a local community occurred from a polyvinyl manufacturer in Minamata, where the evidence for methyl mercury poisoning was absolutely indisputable and resulted in birth defects, among others.[56] Methyl mercury, the form of mercury which can easily be absorbed by humans, largely occurs when rivers are dammed. When trees die and decompose in the waterbed, methylating micro-organisms release the elemental mercury from soil and rock under the waterbed and transform it into this organic form of mercury which is more dangerous for humans. The more hydro dams in an area, the more methyl mercury is created.

---

[54] Sichel, M, *How to Repair Children Damaged by Mercury, Medicine and Politics*, Fountaindale Books, Sydney, 2007, p 147.
[55] Palmer, R.F., et al., Proximity to point sources of environmental mercury release as a predictor of autism prevalence. Health & Place (2008), doi: 10.1016/j.healthplace.2008.02.001.
[56] Smith, R & Lourie, B, *Slow Death by Rubber Duck,* University of Queensland Press, 2009, p 150

The most controversial use of mercury is putting it in vaccinations in the form of thiomersal ('Thiomerosal' in USA). Fortunately, this use has come under the microscope and there have been good efforts to remove it.[57]

Unlike the other toxic elements, mercury is able to cross the blood-brain and the placental barriers.[58] Mercury acts primarily on the neurological system and the gastro-intestinal tract. It can adversely affect developing nerve sheaths by preventing myelin formation.

I have found that mercury, more than other metals, prevents the therapeutic action of well chosen remedies. As recorded in *Boericke*[59], "[e]very organ and tissue of the body is more or less affected by this powerful drug; it transforms healthy cells into decrepit, inflamed and necrotic wrecks...". Patients with mercury are sensitive to any therapeutic intervention. More than other heavy metal patients, they can easily aggravate on many medications, including homeopathic medicine.

Sources
- Coal-fired power plants
- Energy efficient / fluorescent light bulbs
- Fish
- Mercury dental amalgams
- Mercury thermometers,
- Old light switches and thermostats
- Some insecticides and fungicides
- Vaccines containing thiomersol (up to 2002 in Australia).

Toxic Effects
- 'Foggy head'
- 'Leaky gut' with significant food sensitivities
- Anxiety, restlessness
- Any catarrhal irritation of any mucous membrane
- Autistic Spectrum Disorder
- Conduces to infestation with intestinal parasites (helminths, amoebas, etc)
- Dermatitis
- Endocrine disturbance, especially hypothyroidism
- Excessive salivation
- Fatigue
- Gut pain with altered function – "irritable bowel syndrome"
- Headaches
- Inflamed mucous membranes with or without ulceration
- Obsessive compulsive disorder (also Copper)
- Speech or learning delay
- Unresponsive gingivitis.

---

[57] US Centre for Disease Control: "Mercury and Vaccines (Thiomersal)" http://www.cdc.gov/vaccinesafety/concerns/thiomersal.htm
[58] Smith & Lourie, op cit, p 154
[59] Boericke, W, *Homeopathic Materia Medica*, 2nd ed, 1990

Provings

The *Provings* of Mercury show an affinity with mucous membrane, the nervous system and lymphatic tissue:

- Caries of bony tissue
- Chills and profuse perspiration
- Diarrhoea with haemorrhage and inflammation
- Sensitivity to temperature fluctuations
- Tremors, chorea with nocturnal aggravation
- Ulceration, inflammation, necrosis of mucous membrane
- Weakness.

Removing Mercury

- Zinc (antagonist)[60]: 1 tablet daily of approximately 30 mg of elemental zinc, if there is an absolute zinc deficiency (below the reference range) Check for zinc deficiency in relation to copper, cadmium and mercury. Relative deficiency requires higher levels of zinc supplementation. With any ongoing supplementation, HTMA's should be checked every 3-6 months to monitor levels.
- Selenium (antagonist): 5 drops of selenium (50µg) daily. This can be increased if the patient has a frank selenium deficiency.
- Coriander as tincture or fresh each day in food. One practitioner places coriander tincture onto a '*Footsie*' foot pad to help remove mercury from children.[61]
- *Mercury chelate* (one bottle containing homeopathic potency chords of *Mercurius sol* 6c, 12c, 30c, 200c): one dose every second day. This may be given in alternation with the *similimum*.

Note: autistic patients do not present reliable Hair Analysis reports as far as mercury is concerned until many months after a chelation treatment. The presence of mercury will initially be understated or absent on the patient's HTMA.[62]

Example

One patient had a post nasal drip for 15 years which was unresponsive to treatment until his mercury amalgams were removed and his tissue mercury was chelated.

---

[60] Gaetke, L, et al, Copper Toxicity, Oxidative Stress and Antioxidant Nutrients, *Toxicology,* 2003 doi:10.1016/j.physletb.2003.10.071
[61] Sichel, M, *How to Repair,* op cit
[62] Sichel, M, *The Sichel Protocol,* Bookbound Publishing, Ourimbah, Australia, 2007, p 2

Example

This 40 year-old man had pain in the right hypochondrium (hepatic region) with "leaky gut" food reactions. His urinalysis showed no heavy metals, but his HTMA told a different story, suggesting his ability to excrete mercury was impaired via liver and urine: his body was only able to excrete it through the hair. All therapies, including traditional homeopathy, were unsuccessful in helping this man. His symptoms, which were unresponsive to any therapy he had tried, were eventually removed by undergoing rapid chelation therapy.

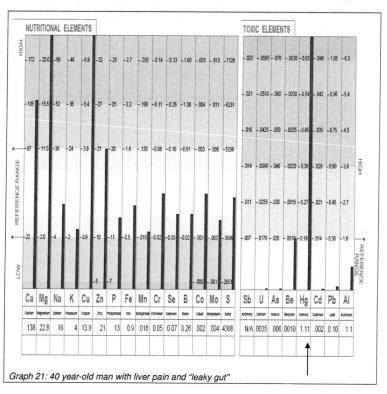

Graph 21: 40 year-old man with liver pain and "leaky gut"

Example

This 30 year old man had gut pain, fatigue, allergies, candida, intestinal parasities and chronic prostatitis. His **serum** mercury was elevated over the reference range, and the graph below shows the mercury revealed in his hair tissue sample *after* 12 months oral of chelation (prior to starting homeopathic treatment).

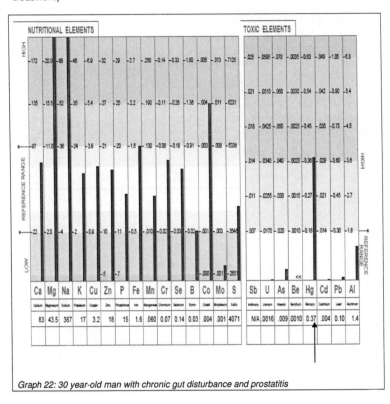

Graph 22: 30 year-old man with chronic gut disturbance and prostatitis

88

Mixed Metal Pictures

Many patients have a multiple heavy metal accumulation. The result is that the neat symptom pictures described above become confused. It is then unclear whether there is a single element, or several elements, which are contributing to the symptoms.

Example
This young girl with high copper, mercury, cadmium, lead and zinc has abdominal pain; chronic loose stools and fatigue.

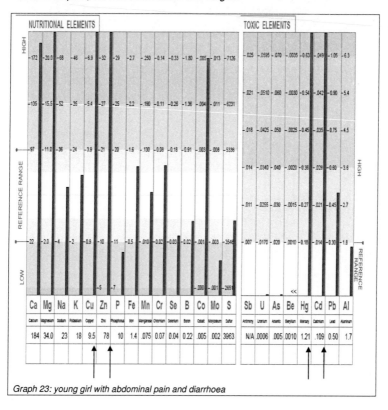

Graph 23: young girl with abdominal pain and diarrhoea

Example

This teenage boy with high copper and cadmium has chronic fatigue, restless limbs, insomnia, recurring viral infections and chronic sinus congestion.

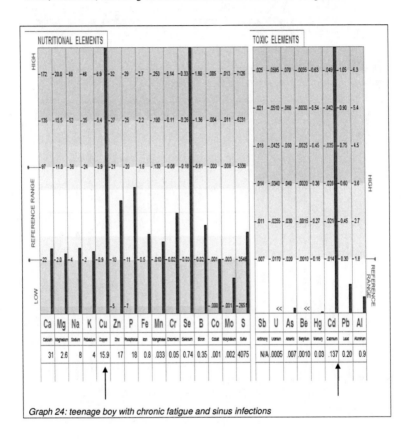

Graph 24: teenage boy with chronic fatigue and sinus infections

Example

This 10 year-old girl had repeated abdominal pain and soiling, urinary tract infections, fatigue and irritability. Her cocktail of high copper and significant amounts of arsenic, cadmium and aluminium were gently chelated with CH77 and minerals over a 12 month period. She was also given a treatment for intestinal parasites.

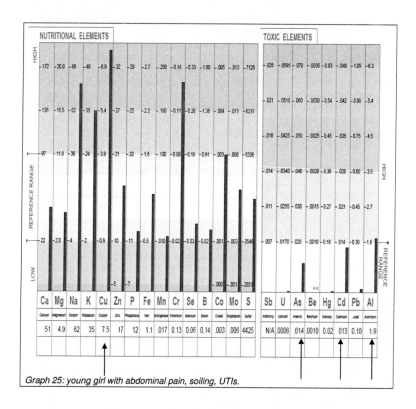

Graph 25: young girl with abdominal pain, soiling, UTIs.

Removing mixed heavy metal accumulations

Remember that our first task as clinicians is to restore the patient to health gently, rapidly and permanently. We must treat the patient, not the toxic metal. Therefore, it is important to choose which, if any, of the toxic elements is likely to be causing the symptoms. It may be possible to do this by reference to the toxic element pictures in this chapter. For example, fatigue with restlessness is likely to be copper related. Fatigue with sluggishness is more likely to be cadmium or lead related.

In confused symptom pictures, we may not be able to decide which, if any, toxic element is foremost as the cause of symptoms. In these cases it is better to give general chelation treatment, using a product such as *CH77*, in addition to the homeopathic remedy of choice. Here are some treatment plan possibilities:

- Choose the metal which is producing the strongest symptom picture and give that in the multiple potency metal formula. Eg to the teenage boy with insomnia, fatigue and recurring sinus infections (see Graph 24), I gave *Copper Chelate*, one dose every second day.
- On the alternate day to the homeopathic chelation one can give the *simillimum*. See Case 6 in Chapter 9, to whom I gave *China sulph 30c* on the alternate day.
- Use a gentle general chelation agent at the same time, such as *CH77*. Be sure that the patient's saliva pH is close to 7.0, as described in the previous chapter (alkalinity assists chelation).
- If it is not known which single toxic element is causing the symptoms, it is better to prescribe only a general chelation agent, such as *CH77*, in addition to the remedy of choice. In the case example shown in Graph 19, I used *CH77* as the main chelation treatment, prescribing individual remedies as needed. This is because the patient, a woman whose hair was coloured, did not eventually send a hair sample for analysis until four months into treatment. I knew there was a strong presence of heavy metal toxicity from her urine test, but I did not know which one when I commenced treatment: thus I used a general chelation agent to cover all heavy metals. This however, is neither specific nor as rapid as using the homeopathic chelation method.
- In addition, give the nutritional elements, zinc and selenium, which antagonises the heavy metals, especially where these are deficient: zinc and selenium.

Therapeutic Summary

Obstacle	Treatment
Toxic elements: cadmium	Cadmium chelate: 1 dose every 2nd day
	Zinc: 30mg elemental zinc per day
Toxic element: excess copper	Copper chelate: 1 dose every 2nd day
	Zinc: 30mg elemental zinc per day
Toxic element: lead	Lead Chelate: 1 dose every 2nd day
	Check calcium and iron for antagonistic activity
Toxic element: mercury	Mercury chelate: 1 dose every 2nd day
	Zinc: 30mg elemental zinc daily
	Selenium: 50µg daily (caution taking selenium for long periods)
Mixed metal accumulations	General chelation agents and appropriate nutritional supplements

Paraphrased from the Organon, Aphorisms 74-75

More particularly in recent times, chronic diseases commonly met,
produced by artificial use of toxic substances, are the most incurable, and it
is impossible to discover any remedies for their cure...

Chapter 6
Chemical Toxicity

If heavy metals, which are naturally occurring elements, are hidden sources of toxicity, then modern man-made chemicals present even more obscure, yet no less toxic, obstacles to cure.

Chemical toxicity is a new health challenge and should be suspected in chronic diseases that are not responding to treatment. No studies are being done on the cumulative effects of chemicals, particularly on babies and young children. Since I have been targeting chemical toxicity with the methods in this chapter, more of the obstinate cases are improving.

Petro-chemical based substances, the extent and reach of which is vast and inescapable, did not exist in the 18th century. There are over 80,000 synthetic chemicals in daily use; in horticulture, farming, food production and processing. At home, they are found in everyday products, like plastics and packaging, cleaning products, garden chemicals, baby bottles, food cans, stain treatments, body care products and cleansers. When you consider that multiple chemicals (some sources report up to 300) are found in breast milk,[63] [64] one realises the impact that chemicals can have on health.

One may ask – don't governments regulate safety levels? Unfortunately: no. Many of these chemicals are well known and documented as being carcinogens, endocrine disruptors and teratogenic. They are bioaccumulative and indisputably toxic.

When treating patients with chronic illness that is unresponsive to treatment, the possibility of chemical toxicity is ever increasing .The sheer number and classes of chemicals makes it impossible to cover them in a single chapter of this book. Rather, I would like to refer you to some key websites that outline the categories of environmental toxins and the dangers that they pose for human health:
- National Toxics Network http://ntn.org.au/ a community based network working to ensure a toxic-free future for all.
- Environmental Working Group http://www.ewg.org/ a non-profit organisation that aims to use the power of public information to protect public health and the environment.

Many chemicals resist degradation by chemical, physical or biological means. They have persistent half-lives (the time taken for half of the quantity of pesticide to degrade) ranging from months to decades and longer: and so are described as Persistent Organic Pollutants (POP's).[65] POP's do not respect

---

[63] Environmental Toxicology and Pharmacology Volume 18, Issue 3, December 2004, pp 259-266
[64] http://ehpnet1.niehs.nih.gov/members/2002/110pA339-A347solomon/solomon-full.html#summ
[65] http://chm.pops.int/default.aspx

international boundaries: they circulate the world in cloud vapour and descend when it rains. POP's are washed into the water systems and accumulate in the fatty tissue of marine life – and eventually those that eat it. Organic food producers cannot avoid exposure to POP's and patients may believe that they have had no exposure to POP's at any time in their life.

Everyone has exposure, no matter where they live and how pure their lifestyle. In 2008, one Canadian researcher tested his own bloodstream for the presence of a POP called *Hexachlorobenzene,* a toxic fungicide which had been banned in his country in the 1970s. Despite no known contact with this chemical, he tested positive at 1.2ng/mLμ[66]

It is the *amount of exposure to and the individual susceptibility* to chemicals that will determine the effect in each patient and their offspring.

To get some idea of the array and effects of POP's, see the *Stockholm Convention's* website on Persistent Organic Pollutants: http://chm.pops.int/. The Stockholm Convention is a global treaty to protect human health and the environment from environmental pollutants and makes recommendations for reducing exposure to governments around the world. The Convention is based in Geneva, Switzerland and administered by the United Nations Environment Programme. At least 172 countries are ratified with the Convention and have national implementation plans in various stages of development.

Becoming aware of the range and health effects of environmental chemicals, leads us to broaden our view when taking our chronically ill patients' cases.

---

[66] Smith, R & Lourie, B, *Slow Death by Rubber Duck,* QUP, 2008, p 193

Some Examples of Household Chemicals

Item	Chemical	Health effects
Plastic food containers: baby bottles, water bottles, food wrapped in plastic or in plastic storage	Bisphenol-A Phthalate	Xenoestrogen, endocrine disruptor carcinogen: breast cancer, infertility, precocious puberty, prostate enlargement
Pesticide residues on food	Organophosphates; organochlorides; carbamates	Xenoestrogen, endocrine disruptor carcinogen, teratogenic, Cholinesterase inhibitor: Cancer, neurological diseases, skin diseases, fatigue
Processed meat	Nitrates 249-252	Methemoglobinaemia (blue baby syndrome); carcinogen, allergy
Herbicides	As for pesticides: other possible chemicals are copper; glyphosate	Xenoestrogen
Cosmetics Sunscreens Antibacterial soaps	Parabens, dioxins, 4-Methylbenzylidene camphor (4-MBC); Methyl 2,3,4	Carcinogen, allergy or sensitivity reactions

Entering the universe of man-made chemicals is overwhelming. So I find it useful to draw a line down the middle: first there are the chemicals whose toxicity to humans and the environment is acknowledged: we try to keep these out of our homes. I have called these 'Toxic Chemicals'. The second are those whose toxicity is not usually acknowledged: these are in our food, personal care products and household cleaners. I have called these 'Benign' Household Chemicals.

1. Toxic Chemicals

Organochloride, Organophosphate & Carbamate Pesticides (POP's)
The organophosphates are a class of chemicals that are descendants of the original nerve gas used in the World War Two. The common brand names are *Dursban, Diazinon, Parathion* and *Malathion.*

The most infamous of the organochlorides, *DDT,* which was replaced by *Chlordane,* was used from the 1940s to the mid 1980s to treat millions of homes all over the world for insect infestations. No one knows if the house they live in has been treated or not: you cannot smell or see this chemical. Only its accumulated toxic effects can be experienced.

Most of these organochloride pesticides and herbicides have been banned in the western world.[67] Some brand names are *Heptachlor, Chlordane, Aldrin, Dieldrin, Lindane* and *Endrin.*

---

[67] A brief summary of these chemicals can be found in Rapp, Dr D, *Our Toxic World, A Wake-Up Call,* Environmental Medical Research Foundation, NY, 2004 from which I make judicious quotes

Examples of exposure and toxicity

- *2,4-D*, a selective weed killer, is still used in Australia: the reason why golf courses are so green and weed-free, now you know why.
- *Lindane* was used until recently as a treatment for head lice.
- *Endosulphan*, a toxic organochloride is still legal in Australia despite its ban in 27 EEC countries, is found in human breast milk.[68]
- In 2008, one Canadian researcher tested his own bloodstream for the presence of another POP, *Hexachlorobenzene,* a fungicide that had been banned in his country in the 1970s. Despite no known contact with this chemical, he tested positive at 1.2 ng/mL[69]
- Children of mothers who used an organophosphate flea shampoo (*eg Dichlorvos*) on their pets during pregnancy have double the chance of developing a brain tumour before the age of five years.[70]
- Prenatal or infant exposure to pest strips increases the risk of leukaemia in young children.[71]
- *2-4-D* and *Lindane* are implicated in the increase of lymphoma and other cancers; *2-4-D* has caused innumerable health problems, typical of pesticide poisoning and chemical sensitivities, not only in the Vietnamese but in the Vietnam War veterans *and their offspring.*
- *Pentachlorophenol (PCP)* is used as an outdoor wood or patio preservative. It was banned in Germany for indoor use after people developed nervous system disease and psychological problems after using it.
- *Polychlorinated or Brominated Biphenols (PCBs and PBBs)* are found in transformers and electrical equipment and are major worldwide sources of PCBs.[72] They are carcinogenic and damage the liver, skin and blood. They affect the immune, reproductive and nervous systems. Research has shown that in time, developmental delays and learning problems are typical.[73] In one study, exposed pregnant mothers had sons with smaller than normal penises.[74]
- *Carbon tetrachloride, Trichloroethylene and Perchloroethylene,* are found in paint, dry cleaning solution and degreasing agents are cleaning products. They can cause confusion, sleepiness, anaesthesia and sometimes death. They contributed to the health complaints of the 'Love Canal' victims in Massachusetts where it was found in their water supply, having been dumped into the waterways for 11 years by a plastic manufacturer.[75]

---

[68] http://www.smh.com.au/environment/study-puts-pesticides-safety-in-spotlight-once-again-20090920-fwsw.html
[69] Smith, R & Lourie, B, *Slow Death by Rubber Duck,* QUP, 2008, p 193
[70] Steinman, D & Wisner, R, *Living Health in a Toxic World,* Berkley Publishing Group, New York, NY, 1995
[71] Ibid
[72] Sherman, J M, MD, *Chemical Exposure and Disease: Diagnostic and Investigative Techniques,* 1994, Princeton Scientific Publishing; Colborn, T, Dumanski, D and Peterson Myres, J, *Our Stolen Future: Are We Threatening our Fertility, Intelligence and Survival?* Penguin Books, NY, 1996
[73] Colborn, et al, ibid
[74] Ibid
[75] Rapp, ibid

- *Diazinon,* banned in Australia only a decade ago, was used routinely in home vegetable gardens. It causes headaches, nausea, dizziness, blurred vision and memory loss. In animals it has shown to cause decrease in coordination, birth defects, stillbirths and a delay in sexual development. In humans it has been associated with an increased risk of brain cancer in children and non-Hodgkin's lymphoma in farming communities in Minnesota and Nebraska.[76] Despite its ban for domestic use, this chemical is still used in agricultural production, as sheep dip. Might this explain patients who have sensitivity reactions to wool?

Health Effects of Organochlorides
- Cancers
- Confusion, aggression or bizarre behaviour
- Developmental delay
- Headaches
- Hypotonia
- Kidney damage in acute exposures
- Memory loss
- Muscle weakness and peripheral neuropathy
- Seizures
- Tachycardia
- Tremor
- Xenoestrogenic effects.

Health Effects of Organophosphates
Organophosphates pesticides interfere with the proper functioning of the nervous system by inhibiting the breakdown of acetylcholine. If it is not broken down, acetylcholine accumulates and begins to impair normal nerve conduction so that nerve impulses are not properly transmitted throughout the body. This class of chemicals is therefore often described as 'Cholinesterase inhibitors'. Like their cousins, the organophosphates are also carcinogens.

Safe Limits
There is much ignorance about 'safe' limits of chemicals and their degree of persistence. In Chapter 10 I discuss a patient who, having recovered from cancer, was spraying his vegetables regularly. I prescribed the *Pesticide, Herbicide & Fungicide Protocol* (described at the end of this chapter) for detoxification, after which his monthly relapse of skin cancers suddenly stopped and he remains in good health to this day. I realised from this and other cases that so many of our patients with chronic illnesses could have these chemical residues as obstacles to cure. To restore health, chemicals have to be removed. It is for this reason that I have begun using the *tautopathic* potencies of these chemicals in a methodical way with certain patients. They can and must be removed in a targeted and specific way as part of the treatment plan.

---

[76] Cox, C, "Carbaryl", Journal of Pesticide Reform, Spring 1993: 13 (1), Northwest Coalition for Alternatives to Pesticides, Eugene:
http://panna.igc.org/resources/pestis/PESTIS.1996.18.html.

Scientists agree that many chemicals are dangerous once our accumulation exceeds a certain amount. There is no certainty about the 'safe' limit when there is a bio-accumulation of chemicals over a lifetime. However, as homeopaths we know that small amounts of chemicals can also have a *dynamic* effect on patients.

Industrial Chemicals (hydrocarbons)

Hydrocarbons, from the petrol in the fuel tank, to the paint thinner, are highly toxic in 'excessive amounts'. Here are a few of the significant ones:

- *Benzene* is a universal solvent used in engine fuels and in the plastic, paint and textile industries. It can damage bone marrow and, in particular, cause leukemia and bone marrow tumors.[77]

- *Toluene* is used to dissolve many common products, especially printer's ink. It damages the nervous system, liver, kidneys, lungs, skin and eyes and can cause developmental delays children.[78]

- *Xylene* is used in insecticides, plastics, spray paints and inks, as well as in the photography, leather and rubber industries. It can damage the brain, kidneys, eyes, skin and cause numbness of the extremities, as well as cause poor coordination, nausea and dizziness.[79]

---

[77] Rapp, Dr D, *Our Toxic World, A Wake-Up Call,* Environmental Medical Research Foundation, NY, 2004
[78] Rapp, ibid
[79] Rapp, ibid

(1) At a Glance: Common Toxic Chemicals

Chemical	Comment
2,4-D & 2-4-5-T	'Agent Orange' widely used in the Vietnam war. Associated with non-Hodgkin's lymphoma, neurological impairment, asthma, immune system suppression, reproductive problems and birth defects.[80]
Alkylphenols	Intermediate chemical used in the manufacture of other chemicals
Atrazine	Weedkiller
Chlordane (oxichlorodane) (derivative of DDT)	Insecticide; acknowledged hormone disruptor
Diazinon	Lice treatment in sheep; used domestically until recent years
Dichlorodiphenyl-dichloroethylene	A breakdown product of DDT; hormone disruptor
Dieldrin (derivative of DDT)	Insecticide and hormone disruptor.
DDE (byproduct of DDT)	Insecticide, carcinogen (eg prostate cancer); developmental toxin; hormone disruptor; respiratory toxin
DDT	Insecticide and carcinogen
Endosulfan	Insecticide still legal in Australia despite its ban in the EEC
Heptachlor	Insecticide, carcinogen; hormone disruptor
Hexachlorobenzene	Fungicide; carcinogen; hormone disruptor and developmental toxin
Lindane	Insecticide; carcinogen; neurotoxin; hormone disruptor
Nonylphenol & derivatives	Industrial surfactants, emulsifiers for emulsion polymerisation; laboratory detergents; pesticides
Pentachlorophenol	General biocide and wood preservative
Polychlorinated biphenyls (PCBs)	In electrical oils, lubricants, plastics, adhesives, paints; very persistent despite their ban decades ago.

A list of the common pesticides, herbicides and fungicide chemicals is in Appendix 4.

---

[80] Cox, C, "2,4-D Toxicology: Part 2", Journal of Pesticide Reform 19, no 2, Summer 1999.

Common Household Chemicals

Product	ingredient
Ant killer	Dieldrin
Blackberry spray	2-4-5-T; 2-4-D
Cabbage Dust	Lindane or DDT
Cockroach bomb	Chlordane; Heptachlor
Ear Drops (Veterinary)	Lindane
Flea Shampoo	Dieldrin, Lindane
Fly spray	Lindane or DDT
Personal Insect Repellant	Hexachlorophene
Rose Dust	Lindane
Seed Dressing	Lindane
Sheep or cattle dip	Lindane; Dieldrin
Snail and slug killer	Lindane
Termite spray	Chlordane, Heptachlor, Dieldrin
Tomato dust	DDT
Vegetable Dust	DDT, Lindane
Wood preservative	Pentachlorophenol
Wood Preserving Oil	Pentachlorophenol

2: 'Benign' household chemicals

Household chemicals are *under-estimated*, and may be a greater threat to health, because we are continually exposed to them and are largely unaware of the health effects that they have.

Household chemicals are of more concern because their toxicity is not officially acknowledged, despite overwhelming evidence from science. These 'benign' chemicals are in body care products, plastic ware and Teflon cookware. The plastic baby bottle probably contains *Bisphenol A* (banned in Canada and several states in USA in 2008) [81] It is likely you have something toxic in your skin cream, even if it says 'natural' on the packet. Even toothpaste contains Triclosans, which turn into dioxins when they reach the water ways.

Chemicals have official 'safe limits', but that limit ignores the bio-accumulation of a broad spectrum of these chemicals in human tissue. Most scientists are unaware about the *dynamic* sensitivity to POP's. Dr Fred von Saal, a professor at the University of Missouri, found this alarming result with *Bisphenol A (BPA)*: "...[W]e demonstrated that a dose of *BPA* 25,000 times lower that had ever been tested also stimulated prostate development exactly like low doses of *oestradiol*. This had been missed in the high-dose [BPA]

---

[81] On 30 June 2010 the Australian Government announced an industry agreement to stop using Bisphenol A in the manufacture of baby bottles

studies." In other words, there is a homeopathic effect from exposure to micro doses of chemicals of which *BPA* is one example. In the words of another source: it causes cell hyperplasia even at 0.025 iug/kg, which is far below the acknowledged 'toxic' dose.[82] This was recently demonstrated in regard to prostate cancer, where nano-particles of *BPA* were able to stimulate carcinogenic activity.[83]

Xenoestrogens

Xenoestrogens are man-made chemicals which exert an oestrogenic influence on human (and animal) tissue. While there is growing evidence of the oncogenetic affect of xenoestrogens, specifically in relation to breast cancer,[84] it is now widely accepted that xenoestrogens are endocrine and reproductive disruptors. "Life relies on the transmission of biochemical information to the next generation, and the presence of xenoestrogens may interfere with this transgenerational information process through chemical confusion."(Vidaeff and Sever[85]).

Tissue hyperplasia and cancer

Xenoestrogens are responsible for oestrogenic effects on certain tissue, especially breast, uterus and prostate. Benign and malignant hyperplasia of these tissues is increasing at an alarming rate. This includes breast, ovary, uterine and prostate hyperplasias and cancer. Prostate cancer has increased by 300% in the last decade. *Bisphenol A* is now acknowledged as a cause of prostate cancer.[86]

Precocious puberty

Early puberty, especially in girls, is now regarded as a direct result of xenoestrogen accumulation. One parent stated that her bottle-fed baby had started developing pubic hair. Her paediatrician told her it was likely to be caused by the *Bisphenol A* in her plastic baby bottle. When she changed to a *Bisphenol*-free bottle, the pubic hair growth stopped! The more exposure to the plasticisers when young the greater the potential impact later in life.

---

[82] Smith, R & Lourie, B, *Slow Death by Rubber Duck, op cit.*

[83] *Mol Cancer Ther* May 2002,1; 515 http://mct.aacrjournals.org/content/1/7/515.full

[84] Pugazhendhi D, Sadler AJ, Darbre PD (2007). "Comparison of the global gene expression profiles produced by methylparaben, n-butylparaben and 17beta-oestradiol in MCF7 human breast cancer cells". *J Appl Toxicol* 27 (1): 67–77. doi:10.1002/jat.1200. PMID 17121429.
Buterin T, Koch C, Naegeli H (August 2006). "Convergent transcriptional profiles induced by endogenous estrogen and distinct xenoestrogens in breast cancer cells". *Carcinogenesis* 27 (8): 1567–78. doi:10.1093/carcin/bgi339. PMID 16474171.
Darbre PD (March 2006). "Environmental oestrogens, cosmetics and breast cancer". *Best Pract. Res. Clin. Endocrinol. Metab.* 20 (1): 121–43. doi:10.1016/j.beem.2005.09.007. PMID 16522524.
Darbre PD, Aljarrah A, Miller WR, Coldham NG, Sauer MJ, Pope GS (2004). "Concentrations of parabens in human breast tumours". *J Appl Toxicol* 24 (1): 5–13. doi:10.1002/jat.958. PMID 14745841.

[85] Vidaeff AC, Sever LE (2005). "In utero exposure to environmental estrogens and male reproductive health: a systematic review of biological and epidemiologic evidence". *Reprod. Toxicol.* 20 (1): 5–20.

[86] *Mol Cancer Ther* May 2002,1; 515 http://mct.aacrjournals.org/content/1/7/515.full

Cross-sensitisation

Another phenomenon which has emerged is cross-sensitisation. Repeated exposure to certain chemicals can result in a sensitivity reaction to one chemical as well as all its chemical cousins, making life difficult for some patients, since those cousin chemicals are widespread.

An example lies in the common hair colour preparations. Every two months your patient might be applying this chemical cocktail to their scalp. What's in it? *Para-Phenylenediamine (PPD)*. Derived from coal tar, it is found in most hair dye. This petroleum product is also found in rubber, photo developer, oil, ink, textile dyes and dark cosmetics. It is one of the toxic cross-sensitisation chemicals. *PPD* can cause sensitisation dermatitis and asthma. Despite the official caution about skin contact, it is legal to place it in hair dye. Most hair dye comes into contact with the scalp for at least 30 minutes, so can be well absorbed through the skin.

Common allergic reactions are dermatitis of the eyes, ears, scalp and face, rash, extreme swelling and a severe burning sensation on the scalp. Yet a more serious reaction occurs if cross-sensitisation takes place, making your patient sensitive to most textile dyes, pen ink, gasoline, oil, food dyes, medication dyes, preservatives (*Parabens*) and some drugs (all 'caine' drugs (*Benzocaine, Novacaine*), S*ulfonamides, Sulfones, Sulfa* drugs, and *Para-aminobenzoic acid (PABA)*). Perfumes contain 'fragrance' which does not reveal specific ingredients. Trade Practices loopholes permit manufacturers non-disclosure of the ingredients and instead allow generic terms such as 'fragrance', parfum' even 'natural ingredients'. The consumer has no idea what they are applying to their skin... until toxic symptoms develop! If the potential reaction is severe enough to produce anaphylactic symptoms, this means the patient cannot go into public places where s/he has no control over the environment. This is the most severe form of Multiple chemical sensitivity.[87]

(2) At a Glance: Summary of the 'Benign' Chemicals

Plastics

Phthalates	Plasticiser for PVC, used in soft plastics. Found in children's plastic toys, plastic food containers, including lunch wrap and plastic drink bottles. Fortunately, after many years of silent critics over wrapping food in plastic, warnings are starting to appear about wrapping oily food in plastic wrapping (meat, avocado, etc.)
Bisphenol A (BPA)[88]	A polycarbonate used to make hard plastic found in CDs, DVDs, drink bottles, kitchen utensils and appliances; eyeglass lenses, baby bottles, laptop faces.

---

[87] See further: http://www.epa.gov/ttn/atw/hlthef/phenylen.html
[88] On 30 June 2010 the Australian government announced the withdrawal of *Bisphenol A* from the manufacture of baby bottles

Other household chemicals which all have Xenoestrogenic effects

4-Methylbenzylidene camphor (4-MBC)	Sunscreen lotions
Butylated hydroxyanisole (BHA)	Food preservative
Erythrosine	FD & C red No. 3
Ethynylestradiol (combined oral contraceptive pill)	Released into the environment as a xenoestrogen
Metalloestrogens	A class of inorganic xenoestrogens
Parabens	Found in skin lotions
PFCs (perfluorinated compounds)	In non-stick cookware (Teflon), contains perfluorooctanoic acid (PFOA), in pizza boxes, computer mice, cosmetics and clothing. Linked to birth defects, developmental problems, hormone disruption and high cholesterol.[89]
Phenosulfothiazine	Red dye
Propyl gallate	Used to protect oils and fats in products from oxidation
Triclosan	In antibacterial hand soaps, some toothpastes, underwear, some garden hoses, children's toys. Promotes bacterial resistance. Found in breastmilk.[90] Effects: thyroid disturbance, neurological disturbance androgenic effects.[91]

When to expect chemical toxicity

Exposure to these chemicals is therefore a likely factor in patients who have:

- Auto-immune diseases including cancer
- Chronic Fatigue Syndrome and fibromyalgia
- Endocrine diseases
- Neurological diseases
- Reproductive diseases including infertility and precocious puberty (discussed below)
- Sensitisation illnesses including Multiple chemical sensitivity
- Undiagnosable, chronic illnesses.

With the increasing complexity of chemical infiltration into human tissue, we can expect to see more chronically ill patients. Saturation exposure to chemicals can occur through many portals:

- In utero via active exposure
- Trans-placental through prior exposure of the parent
- Use of the 'safe' chemicals described above
- Within patient's lifespan through endogenous exposure, eg breast milk

---

[89] See Danish Environmental Protection Agency, Survey of Chemical Substances in Consumer products, no 99, Sevey & Environmental Health Assessment of Fluorinated Substances in Impregnated Consumer Products and Impregnating Agents (Oct 2008), reported in *Slow Death by Rubber Duck,* op cit.

[90] Allmyr, M, "Triclosan in Plasma and Milk from Swedish Nursing Mothers and Their Exposure via Personal Care Products", Science of the Total Environment 372, no 1 (2006): 87-93

[91] Foran, C, et al, "Developmental Evaluation of a Potential Non-steroidal Estrogen: Triclosan", Marine Environmental Research 50 (2000): 153-56

- Within patient's lifespan via environmental exposure (often resulting in acute illness) or in tiny traces through agricultural insecticides.

Who is most susceptible?

First, people most susceptible are likely to have deficiency in at least two of their antioxidant minerals; specifically zinc and selenium. Both minerals protect against free radical damage, discussed in Chapters 4 and 5. In those chapters I discuss how zinc deficiency in particular causes retention of copper. Patients with high copper will accumulate xenoestrogens more rapidly than those with normal copper. This is because xenoestrogens bind to copper.[92] Xenoestrogens are in both the toxic and 'benign' chemicals.

Finding the chemicals

Conventional blood and urine testing, and Hair Tissue Mineral Analysis, will fail to reveal any of these toxicities. Specialised blood and urine tests need to be used to identify the presence and amount of chemicals. These tests are expensive, and cover only a small group of common agricultural and industrial chemicals. If the chemical to which the patient was exposed is not one of the specific chemicals in the reference group, testing yields no results. Similarly if the exposure was many years ago, it is unlikely to be evident in a blood sample.

The patient's history can reveal an exposure to a known toxic chemical. One case, a patient with a long history of asthma, eczema and dermatitis, had worked at a steel works where he regularly came into contact with a range of hazardous chemicals. His level of exposure was so extreme, that kinesiology muscle testing against potentised samples of various chemicals, exhausted him for days.

A woman who presented with multiple chemical sensitivity told of her husband, who had died of cancer, working in a manufacturing plant for the *Agent Orange* chemical *2-4-D,* the defoliant used during the Vietnam War. She had not made a connection between his exposure and her illness, despite the fact she was living with him for some 15 years during that exposure, when she washed his clothes, slept with him and shared food with him. As well as multiple chemical sensitivity, she had developed Hashimoto's thyroiditis and coeliac disease. This illustrates how we are benumbed, to both the toxicity and the persistence of these chemicals.

Treatment

All of us, no matter how pure our lifestyle, are in some way exposed to some of the chemicals in the above table. Understood in this context, it becomes meaningless to rule out exposure to POP's for any patient. They are a possibility in any serious chronic disease. Therefore I give one, two or all

---

[92] Watts, D, *Trace Elements and other Essential Nutrients,* Writers Block, USA, 1995, p 84

three of the protocols listed below, depending on the disease of the patient and their degree of illness.

Questions to ask in case taking

The area they grew up in. Was there any crop spraying or use of other agricultural chemicals? Nearby coal fired power station, industry?
What were the occupations of family members? What chemicals do they habitually use?
These include:

- Cleaning products
- Garden chemicals/sprays
- History of fumigating the house
- Household insect sprays/pest strips
- Personal care products – look for 'fragrance', 'parfum' on labels
- Plastics use in food storage and preparation
- Teflon/non-stick cookware.

Nutritional needs prior to homeopathic intervention, to assist elimination

- Potential xenoestrogenic effects are amplified if the patient has a zinc deficiency. Based on HTMA, correct the zinc: copper ratio. This is discussed in Chapter 2.
- Make sure their selenium is within the appropriate nutrient range. Again, the HTMA gives the most reliable assay of cellular selenium: see Appendix 2.

Give concurrent liver drainage therapy. Toxins are stored in the liver or removed from tissue via the lymphatics to the liver.
Start drainage with only 1 drop doses of tincture in highly sensitive patients.

Liver Drainage
Herbal tinctures 1:2 strength:
- *Greater celandine (chelidonium)* if there is nausea and digestive disturbance (15 drops 3 x daily); or
- *St Mary's thistle*, same dose, particularly if there is liver pathology such as fatty liver; or
- *Dandelion root*, same dose as *St Mary's Thistle*.

Two Homeopathic Treatment Options for Eliminating Chemicals

Here are the three protocols, each of which contains *tautopathic* potencies of the chemicals described. These options can be used for patients even if they have no known exposure to chemicals, since subtle chemical exposure is now universal.

Option 1: *Tautopathy*

Example: woman of 45

This woman worked with the chemical 2,4-D for 15 years. During this time many of her symptoms began: multiple chemical sensitivity, to perfumes and household cleaning products; Hashimoto's thyroiditis; recurring sinusitis and other respiratory infections; coeliac disease.

She received traces of the chemicals in a variety of ways: through intimate contact, and washing her husband's clothes, etc.

Treatment:
- *Day 1: 2,4-D 200c – 3 doses*
- *Day 2: 2,4-D 30c – 3 doses*
- *Day 3: 2,4-D 16c – 3 doses*

When she took the first dose she reported 'the strong taste of herbicide in her mouth for many hours' followed by diarrhoea and weakness. In herself she felt well, her sleep was peaceful. Once the aggravation passed her chemical sensitivity was much improved.

The aggravation from the *tautopathic* prescription was expected and is a good sign, provided that the aggravation is not too strong for an already frail patient.

However there are two problems with this treatment plan: first we may not be able to ascertain *which chemical* the patient has been exposed to, with no clear history available, or there may be a history of exposures to *many different* chemicals.

When I sourced many of these toxic chemicals some years ago, I did not realise how much I would be using them now. A lab has obliged and potentised these substances for the three distinct detoxifying protocols.

It is impossible to know which chemicals underpin a patient's chronic disease, but we can choose the protocol(s) based on the presenting symptoms. Some patients with intractable chronic disease may benefit from *all three* protocols. Give one protocol over seven days, a different potency each day, first going *down* the potency scale to minimise aggravation, then returning up the potency scale. If an aggravation occurs, stop and wait, then resume the when symptoms have settled. Repeat the protocol several times if needed, depending on the patient's sensitivity and response. The three protocols are listed on the next pages.

Patients can experience these symptoms during treatment:
- 'Chemical' taste or perverted taste sense
- Diarrhoea or vomiting
- Fatigue
- Headache
- Nausea.

1: Pesticide, Herbicide & Fungicide Protocol
A complex of some 120 organochlorides and organophosphates, including *2,4-D, DDT, 2-4-5-t, Lindane, Chlordane, Dieldrin, Endosulphan, Diazinon*

Pesticide, Herbicide & Fungicide Protocol 200c: 3 doses on Day 1.
Pesticide, Herbicide & Fungicide Protocol 30c: 3 doses on Day 2.
Pesticide, Herbicide & Fungicide Protocol 16c: 3 doses on Day 3.
No medicine on Day 4.
Pesticide, Herbicide & Fungicide Protocol 16c: 3 doses on Day 5
Pesticide, Herbicide & Fungicide Protocol 30c: 3 doses on Day 6.
Pesticide, Herbicide & Fungicide Protocol 200c: 3 doses on Day 7.

Dose for all three protocols
Three potencies are given over a 7-day period. The sensitivity of the patient and the degree to which the chemicals have produced the patient's symptoms will determine the level of aggravation experienced by the patient. Giving the descending potencies first lessens the likelihood and degree of aggravation.[93] Although we can think of these symptoms as aggravations in the typical sense, since we are using *tautopathy* (the same) rather than *similia* (similar) it may be more appropriate to describe them as signs that the chemical residues are leaving the body. Patients will understand that their discomfort is a 'detoxification effect' rather than a worsening of their illness. In any event, the patient can pause the protocol if feeling unwell and resume once symptoms have settled.

I give this protocol to some cancer patients, in addition to other 'pathological' prescribing or the *simillimum*. Severe cases can be given all three of the protocols at different times, especially patients with malignancy or Multiple chemical sensitivity. These protocols are an adjunct to the treatment plan: they do not replace the well chosen homeopathic prescription. They do no more than remove potential obstacles to cure.

Protocol 2 is used for detoxifying hydrocarbons and other industrial chemicals for patients with Multiple chemical sensitivity, leukaemia or other blood disorders: such as leukopaenia, thrombocytopaenia and aplastic anaemia.[94]

2: Industrial Chemical Protocol
This protocol contains potentised hydrocarbons, benzene, toluene, xylene, chemicals in hair colourings, nail varnishes, paint removers, etc:

Industrial Chemical Protocol 200c: 3 doses on Day 1
Industrial Chemical Protocol 30c: 3 doses on Day 2.
Industrial Chemical Protocol 16c: 3 doses on Day 3
No medicine on Day 4
Industrial Chemical Protocol 16c: 3 doses on Day 5
Industrial Chemical Protocol 30c: 3 doses on Day 6
Industrial Chemical Protocol 200c: 3 doses on Day 7.

---

[93] Cole, J & Dyson, R, Classical Homeopathy Revisited, UK, after the work of Pritnam Singh.
[94] http://www.atsdr.cdc.gov/csem/benzene/physiologic_effects.html

3: Xenoestrogen Protocol
For patients with hormonal symptoms, precocious puberty, reproductive hyperplasia and unexplained infertility. Contains potentised samples of plasticisers, and chemicals from plastic manufacture, plus synthetic oestrogens etc
Xenoestrogen Protocol 200c: 3 doses on Day 1
Xenoestrogen Protocol 30c: 3 doses on Day 2
Xenoestrogen Protocol 16c: 3 doses on Day 3
No medicine on Day 4
Xenoestrogen Protocol 16c: 3 doses on Day 5
Xenoestrogen Protocol 30c: 3 doses on Day 6
Xenoestrogen Protocol 200c: 3 doses on Day 7.

Option 2: Antidote / Antipsoric
This second method is only recommended where:
- A patient with chemical sensitivity has not responded to the above protocol, and/or
- Constitutional prescribing has been unsuccessful

This is a more gentle treatment approach than Option 1 and is less likely to cause aggravation. However, because it is less specific in its therapeutic reach, containing no *tautopathic* ingredients, it needs to be given for much longer for it to reach a deep-seated chemical obstacle to cure. The patient may have to continue the treatment below for many months or years. Nor is it always successful in terms of clearing disease symptoms. Yet it may clarify disease symptoms so that a new homeopathic prescription may become clear in time.

Prescribe *Camphor 200c*, 1 dose once every second day. On the alternate day give an *anti-miasmatic* remedy based on the patient's generals. Most patients will need an *antipsoric* remedy, because most of the symptom presentations are functional disturbances: eg skin irritations, asthma, sinusitis, gastro-intestinal disturbances. Chilly patients have *Psorinum*; hot patients have *Sulphur*. If using *Sulphur*, do not give a decimal or centesimal potency since aggravations can be nasty. Start *Sulphur* with an LM potency of at least LM 0/5. This protocol must be given *for a least three months* before any tangible results will be seen.

This approach has unstuck some of my most difficult cases. My understanding is that *Sulphur*, with its solid reputation as an *antipsoric*, is able to bring to the surface deeply sequestered chemicals. Once those chemicals have been brought to the surface, the *Camphor* antidotes the toxic effects that come with them.

Example
This 47 year-old man had lifelong dermatitis, asthma, sinusitis, frontal headaches, with worsening fatigue and displayed Multiple chemical

sensitivity. He was also allergic to cat fur, dust mites and some pollens. He always felt the heat and all symptoms were aggravated by work stress.

Treatment:
- *Camphor 200c – one dose every 2nd day*
- *Sulphur LM 0/5 – one dose on each alternate day.*

This treatment was continued for 24 months, using increasing potencies of Sulphur LM. he experienced gradual improvement in all symptoms. After 24 months he was symptom free, with virtually no aggravation from his usual allergy triggers.

I recommend *Sulphur* because of its reputation as a detoxifier both as a homeopathic remedy and as a bio-mineral. Remember; give this treatment for at least three months before expecting any tangible results.

In Conclusion
Chemical exposure and toxicity is an overwhelming area of bioscience. A small amount of key information is helpful to our understanding of what may be affecting our patients.

Also important is to educate ourselves and our patients on avoiding chemical exposure. Phenomenal efforts are being made around the world in this quest.
 The Environmental Working Group is a non-profit organization that offers a lot of information at the press of a button on their website:
 http://www.ewg.org/Health-Tips

The *Health Tips* section offers easy to read, understand and use guides on:

- Avoiding BPA,
- Baby bottles & feeding formulas
- Healthy Home Tips
- PFC's
- Safe Drinking Water,
- Shoppers Guide to avoiding Pesticides
- Sunscreens
- Triclosan

This information is positive and helpful; patients like to know about avoiding chemical if it seems manageable.

Also, refer to the websites listed on the first and second pages of this chapter – the information is vast, detailed and compelling.

Further Reading
Slow Death by Rubber Duck.[95]

---

[95] Smith, R, & Lourie, B, *Slow Death by Rubber Duck: How the Toxic Chemistry of Everyday Life Affects our Health,* University of Queensland Press, 2009

Chapter 7
Iatrogenesis

The term 'iatrogenesis' derives from the Greek *'iatros'* meaning physician, and *'genesis'* meaning beginning.

Treating this case set me on a path of looking for 'exciting causes' from existing allopathic treatments, in greater detail:

A woman in her 70's presented with a gagging cough that she had had for several months. She and her husband were exhausted from lack of sleep. By the time she came to clinic, she was desperate for her cough to stop. I prescribed *Hepar Sulph 200c*, her cough improved quickly and everyone was pleased. Then her cough returned, while still taking the *Hepar Sulph*. I changed the potency to *Hepar Sulph 6c* with a similar result, but her cough returned again. Puzzled as to the substantial improvement then relapse, I asked her if she was taking anything that might antidote the remedy at the same time. Eventually, her pharmacist recognised that a side effect of her heart medication was laryngeal spasm. Her heart medication was changed, and her cough duly stopped.

I did not take her case thoroughly enough to pinpoint when the cough started in relation to her starting her heart medication. Homeopathy had not failed and the medication was her clear obstacle to cure.

Here are some statistics on side effects from medications:
- The total number of adverse reactions to drugs in Australia from the years 1999 - 2000 (those resulting in hospital admission and those that did not) was 400,000.[96]
- There are 140,000 hospital admissions in Australia every year because of misused pharmaceutical drugs.[97]
- In the US, doctors are the third leading cause of death, with iatrogenic disease accounting for 250,000 deaths every year: I2, 000 from unnecessary surgery, **7,000 from medication errors in hospitals,** 20,000 from other errors in hospitals, 80,000 from infections in hospitals, **106,000 from the negative effects of drugs.**[98]
- In the US up to one fifth of all new prescription drugs may ultimately be recalled or produce potentially harmful side effects.[99]
- Up to 15% of hospital admissions in Europe are due to adverse drug reactions.[100]

---

[96] Australian Journal of Pharmacy, 83, September 2002, 774
[97] Australian Journal of Pharmacy, 83, September 2002, 774
[98] Journal of the American Medical Association, 84, July 26, 2000
[99] Journal of the American Medical Association, 2002; 287:2215-2220, 2273-2275
[100] Australian Journal of Pharmacy, 83, November 2002, 885

All pharmaceutical drugs have the ability to cause iatrogenic symptoms, depending on the dosage and sensitivity of the patient. We need to be familiar with, or access information about the side effects of our patients' medications. Symptoms caused by a medication may not improve until it is discontinued.

Some commonly prescribed drugs that cause multiple side effects are:

Statins (*Lipitor, Zocor*)
Some 36 million Americans take a daily *statin* prescribed for the rest of their lives, which may even be causing the heart conditions they are allegedly preventing.[101]

Statin side effects are:
- Muscle pain: soreness, tiredness or weakness severe enough to make daily activities like climbing stairs or walking difficult.
- Liver damage: can develop without symptoms, resulting in *permanent* liver damage. To prevent this occurrence a monitoring blood test is needed every six weeks to 12 weeks for the first year and every time the *statin* dose is increased.
- *Digestive problems:* nausea, diarrhea or constipation
- *Rash or flushing* which can be aggravated if taken with niacin (vitamin B3)
- *Neurological side effects*: although unconfirmed, research suggests a possible link.[102]

Oral Contraceptive Pill / Copper IUD
The OCP has a long list of side effects, which are important to consider in your patient who may be presenting with a seemingly unrelated illness.
OCP side effects are:
- Acne (or acne is treated *with* the OCP)
- Anxiety
- Cervical dysplasia
- Chloasma
- Depression
- Elevated cholesterol -> gallstones
- Fatigue
- Foggy thinking
- General body aches
- Headaches
- Hypertension
- Insomnia
- Libido decreased
- Monilia thrush
- Nausea
- Premenstrual headache
- Sinusitis
- Weight gain.

---

[101] The Lancet, 2007; 369: 268-9
[102] http://www.mayoclinic.com/health/statin-side-effects/MY00205

The most common presentation I see is vaginal thrush with headaches and mood disturbance. This may be related to an increase in copper levels, which affect mood, sleep and liver function. Synthetic oestrogens cause copper retention and biliary stasis in susceptible individuals. Many of these patients have low zinc - a further reason why copper is retained to toxic levels: see Chapters 2 and 5.

Treatment
The OCP is best discontinued. To antidote the sequelae caused by taking the Pill, give *Folliculinum 30c*, one dose every second day for two to four weeks. If there is high copper, prescribe a zinc and vitamin C supplement. If the copper is very high, due to its association with oestrogen, and there are symptoms present of the type described in Chapter 5 in the *Copper* section, also give *Copper Chelate*, once every second day for weeks to months.

Hormone Replacement Therapy (HRT)
HRT also has far reaching side effects as shown by the well-known US trial that that was halted half way through due to the increased risk of hormonally related cancers. HRT can be considered as an obstacle to cure in unresponsive patients using this range of medications.

Paracetamol
A study of over 200,000 children from 31 countries published in *The Lancet* [103] suggests that using *paracetamol* in the first year of life is linked to an increased risk of asthma and other allergies. The study also found that 6 to 7 year-olds who had taken paracetamol once a month in the 12 months prior had a **had a three fold increase risk of asthma.** This may in part explain the burgeoning incidence of allergies in developed countries. It would be interesting to see if *paracetamol* given tautopathically could benefit unresponsive children who have received large amounts of *paracetamol* in their early years.

An explanation of how this may be possible is that *paracetamol* reduces antioxidant defenses, responsible for to inflammation in the airways; the basis of asthma. It may switch the immune system to become more allergic.

Antibiotics
The far-reaching effects of antibiotic use may not yet be known, but there are some definite areas of iatrogenesis that are well known. When *penicillin* was introduced in the 1940's it saved many lives, but now antibiotics are used for ailments that are capable of resolving themselves. Research shows that children who are given antibiotics in the first year of life are more likely to develop asthma in later years. [104] Three quarters of the body's immune function is generated in the bowel. Anything that affects crucial bowel bacteria, affects immune function.

---

[103] The Lancet, Volume 372, Issue 9643, 20 September 2008-26 September 2008, Pages 1039-1048,
[104] *BMJ* 1998; 317:609-610 http://www.bmj.com/cgi/content/full/317/7159/609

Antibiotics will predispose to gut dysbiosis by reducing the colonies of beneficial gut flora, particularly if two or more courses are given for the same infective episode. People who have Irritable Bowel Syndrome (IBS) often have a history of multiple antibiotic prescriptions. An observable long-term sequelae of antibiotics is chronic intestinal candida. This is a common form of gut dysbiosis, which causes:

* bloating, worse after sugar and starchy carbohydrates
* intestinal, vaginal, rectal or oral thrush (monilia).

Treatment
To treat the sequelae of antibiotics, give either *Penicillinum* or *Amoxicillin 30c*, one dose every second day for two to four weeks. The bowel nosode *Gaertner* is sometimes helpful in restoring normal gut function after heavy antibiotic use.

Treatment for intestinal candida (dysbiosis) is discussed in *The Treatment of Irritable Bowel Syndrome.*[105]

Vaccinosis
Vaccinosis is the most infamous of the iatrogenic diseases and there are a variety of approaches to deal with vaccine side effects.

* J Compton-Burnett first described *vaccinosis* in relation to *Thuja* antidoting the effects.[106]
* Dr Tinus Smits[107] and Dr Isaac Golden[108] respectively have done extensive work in this area.
* A well-researched and balanced account of vaccine damage can be found in Dr Richard Halverson's *The Truth About Vaccines.*[109]

The first signs of potential *vaccinosis* are swelling at the site of injection and fever. However the routine practice of giving *paracetamol* makes these symptoms hard to detect. Richard Halverson suggests sequelae can occur up to nine months after vaccination.[110]

Some cases of *vaccinosis* are compelling and lead to the withdrawal of the vaccine: the *2010 influenza vaccination*, which included *Swine Flu* components, had to be withdrawn from use (in Australia) in children because it caused convulsions and other side effects, including some deaths.[111]

---

[105] Gamble, J *Mastering Homeopathy 2: The Treatment of Irritable Bowel Syndrome,* Karuna Publishing, Australia, 2006
[106] J Compton-Burnett, *Vaccinosis and its Cure by Thuja* (1897) (B Jain imprint)
[107] Tinus Smits, http://www.post-vaccination-syndrome.com/3890/treatment.aspx
[108] Golden, Isaac, *Vaccine Damaged Children: Treatment, Prevention, Reasons,* Isaac Golden Publications, Australia; http://www.post-vaccination-syndrome.com/3890/
[109] Halverson, Dr Richard, *The Truth About Vaccines: How We are Used as Guinea Pigs Without Knowing it,* Gibson Square, London, 2007
[110] Halverson, Dr Richard, *The Truth About Vaccines: How We are Used as Guinea Pigs Without Knowing it,* Gibson Square, London, 2007
[111] http://www.health.nsw.gov.au/publichealth/immunisation/index.asp

Controversy over the *MMR vaccine* since Dr Andrew Wakefield's paper was released[112] has created international headlines for over ten years. Despite the predictable torrent of rebuttal within Wakefield's own profession there is considerable anecdotal evidence to suggest a causal relationship between the *MMR vaccine*, inflammatory bowel disease and autism.[113] It is not an uncommon occurrence for parents to report symptoms in their children after the *MMR vaccination.*

The *Meningococcal* vaccine produces a pseudo-meningitis, with symptoms occurring, particularly at night, within a few days of the vaccination:
- Fever
- Headache
- Piercing scream.

The old *DPT vaccine*, now obsolete in Australia, caused these symptoms in some children:
- Behavioural changes or sleep disturbance
- Frequent waking
- Head banging
- Nocturnal fever
- Noted aggravation or side effect at the time of the vaccination
- Repeated upper respiratory infections including otitis media
- Weight loss (unexplained by other factors).

The new *Gardasil* vaccine for Human Papilloma Virus to prevent cervical cancer has been found to cause neurological disturbance in some patients. As of May 2010 there have been 53 deaths reported in the US.[114]

Here is an excerpt from the Therapeutic Goods Administration website: *Australia was one of the first countries to roll out a national cervical cancer immunisation campaign using Gardasil. Over six million doses of Gardasil have been distributed in Australia. Worldwide, over 61 million doses have been distributed. No vaccine is completely without side-effects, and so adverse events following immunisation are carefully monitored in Australia and regularly reviewed by expert advisory groups. As of 17 June 2010, a total of 1,534 suspected adverse reactions have been reported in Australia following vaccination with Gardasil. The great majority have been mild and common problems such as soreness, swelling, or redness at the injection site. Most of the adverse reactions that have been reported are well recognised and listed in the Gardasil Product Information. Common adverse events reported to date are listed below:[115]*

---

[112] Wakefield, Andrew, *Callous Disregard,* Slyhorse Publishing, USA, 2010
[113] Wakefield, ibid
[114] http://www.cdc.gov/vaccinesafety/vaccines/hpv/gardasil.html
[115] Extract from http://www.tga.gov.au/alerts/medicines/gardasil.htm

Suspected adverse reaction To Gardasil	Number of reports (% of total reports)
Injection site reaction	294 (19.1%)
Headache	316 (20.5%)
Dizziness	214 (13.9%)
Nausea	237 (15.4%)
Fatigue and lethargy	152 (10%)
Fever	148 (9.6%)
Fainting	134 (8.7%)
Generally feeling unwell	123 (8.0%)
Vomiting	123 (8.0%)

Serious side effects from the US Centre for Disease Control's website list:
- *Guillain-Barré Syndrome*
- *Blood Clots* have occurred in the heart, lungs, and legs
- *Deaths in the US: 53.*[116]

In clinic, one 13 year-old girl experienced severe leg spasms, with pins and needles, for many months after her *Gardasil* vaccine, until given the homeopathic antidote. The originator of this vaccine, Professor Ian Frazer, acknowledges that side effects occurred in approximately 1:4000 patients, but said the risk of cervical cancer was a more serious risk than the side effects.

Treatment
Well-selected remedies may not work while *vaccinosis* is present. This means either:
- The *dynamic* effect of the vaccine material continues to exert a morbid influence on the patient
- There is a substance contained in the vaccine that has not been excreted. (Since 2002 the vaccines in Australia have been free from *thiomersal* (a form of mercury).

Drs Tinus Smits[117] and Jean Elmiger[118] respectively, offer approaches that effectively neutralise the effects created by vaccines. In Dr Smits' approach, the patient receives the (*tautopathic*) potentised vaccine that contains vaccine excipients as well as the micro-organism source material to antidote the iatrogenic side effects.

Elmiger uses high potency *nosodes* (generally 10M) of the disease for which the original vaccine was given. This approach, subsequently designated as 'Sequential Homeopathic Treatment', has been developed by Canadian homeopath Dr Rudi Verspoor.[119] Elmiger's approach relies on *similia*, in which

---

[116] http://www.cdc.gov/vaccinesafety/vaccines/hpv/gardasil.html
[117] Smits, Dr T, http://www.post-vaccination-syndrome.com/3890/treatment.aspx
[118] Elmiger, Dr Jean *Rediscovering Real Medicine*, Vega, London, 2001
[119] An Interview with Rudi Verspoor describes his work with sequential therapy http://hpathy.com/homeopathic-interviews/rudi-verspoor/

there will be no vaccine excipients, only potentised disease source material in the form of the *nosode*.

Treatment
Tinus Smits approach
Day 1: Vaccine 30c – 2 doses
Day 2: Vaccine 200c – 2 doses
Day 3: Vaccine 1M – 2 doses
Day 4: Vaccine 10M – 2 doses
(Dr Smits now recommends giving each respective potency *one week* apart, with two doses of each potency given each time.)[120]

If either of these potencies of the vaccine produces any aggravations or symptoms, the protocol is stopped until this passes then resumed where it was postponed. Then one moves up to the next potency.

I have found that in most cases a symptom will arise at some point during this protocol, which is a sign that the original vaccine has created an iatrogenic disease that is now being removed by the potentised vaccines.

There are two confirming signs that a child's ill health has been caused by a vaccination:
• An aggravation or re-appearance of an old symptom
• Sudden improvement in symptoms; after the homeopathic 'antidote' has been given.

Example
This 3 year old boy did not start his vaccination program until 12 months. Following the usual schedule, he therefore did not receive his MMR vaccine until the age of 2 years. After the vaccine was given he stopped talking. Two days after the vaccine he developed abdominal pain. In the next 12 months he developed ongoing colds, ear infections and sore throats, none of which he had experienced prior to MMR vaccination.

I gave him MMR 30c, 200c and 1M (I did not have any 10M potency). After the 1M he had "fluorescent green diarrhoea" and vomiting for a day. His speech suddenly improved and he went through the subsequent winter without any colds or sore throats.

Confused drug pictures
The patient may have been given, or used, many different drugs. It may not be clear what drug has produced the obstacle to cure. One patient had a history of illicit intravenous drug use. She had then been given the methadone program. At some point in her history she had contracted Hepatitis C. None of the usual remedies was able to treat her chronic diarrhoea.

---

[120] http://www.post-vaccination-syndrome.com/3890/treatment.aspx

Treatment
In these cases where there are multiple iatrogenic influences, the use of *Camphor 200c* may be the final draw card in the therapeutic pack. *Camphor* was given once every second day for several months. It antidoted the mixture of drug influences, resulting in the cure of her diarrhoea.

Summary of Iatrogenic Protocols

Obstacle	Treatment
Vaccine sequelae (Smits)	*Vaccine 30c –* 2 doses week 1 *Vaccine 200c –* 2 doses week 2 *Vaccine 1M –* 2 doses week 3 *Vaccine 10M –* 2 doses week 4.
Oral Contraceptive Pill	*Folliculinum 30c –* 1 dose every 2nd day for two weeks.
Antibiotic sequelae	*Penicillin or Amoxicillin 30c,* 1 dose every 2nd day for two weeks Candida treatment if needed[121]
Confused iatrogenic drug pictures	*Camphor 200c –* 1 dose every 2nd day for 2 to 8 weeks.

---

[121] Gamble, J, *Mastering Homeopathy 2: The Treatment of Irritable Bowel Syndrome*, Karuna Publishing, Australia, 2006, p 61.

Chapter 8
New Treatment Possibilities:
Electro-magnetic Radiation

This is a brief mention of treatment possibilities for those patients who, after every effort, remain in poor health.

The hazards of **radiation** are well known. The homeopathic principle is well demonstrated with radiation, since small doses will *destroy* malignant cells, and high exposure can *cause* malignancy.

Non-ionizing radiation 'excites' electrons to a higher state of arousal. It can disturb the normal electrical field of cells. The most recognised exposure to non-ionising radiation is through the use of mobile phones. While there is little agreement on just how harmful mobile phones are to health, judging from the vast number of studies, there is certainly a link between their use and some cancers. [122]

Ionising radiation includes the 'stronger' class of radiation, which has the capacity to damage DNA.

Sources of non-ionising radiation:
* Computers, television, radios, *mobile phones.*
* Electric blanket
* Electric metre box
* Mobile phone transmission towers
* Micro wave oven
* Wireless internet connections.

Electrical fields:
Electric blankets
Electric metre boxes
High voltage power lines.

It is difficult to establish from the case history if electromagnetic radiation is implicated in the presenting illness. One Chronic Fatigue Syndrome patient who had two siblings also suffering from CFS, lived next to an electricity sub-station during their childhood, so in the absence of other explanations for the CFS, one might consider this a possible cause.

The *materia medica* has remedies that acknowledge the effect of electricity, radiation and X-Ray on the human body. At the time of writing we are trialling

---

[122] Mixed Signals on Cell Phones and Cancer Epidemiology: November 2004 - Volume 15 - Issue 6 - pp 651-652 Savitz, David
http://journals.lww.com/epidem/pages/articleviewer.aspx?year=2004&issue=11000&article=0 0002&type=fulltext

the homeopathic remedies listed below in some of our Chronic Fatigue patients.

Potential Treatment Options for Chronic Health Effects from Electro-Magnetic Radiation

Remedy	*Materia Medica*
Radium Bromide	For pain syndromes, such as fibromyalgia
Magnetis Polis Ambo	Burning lancinations; sharp pains as if the bones were broken; headache as if nail were driven into the head.
X-ray	Chronic fatigue syndromes where fatigue, not pain, is the guiding symptom.
Electricitas	Pain syndromes with sensitivity to electrical storms, and peculiar sensations of tingling in the limbs.

Preventative measures
No electrical devices in bedroom especially mobile phones
Make sure not sleeping between a wireless internet connection, or within 3 m of an electricity metre box
Don't use an electric blanket
Keep clear of the microwave oven when in use

Chapter 9
Heavy Metal Case Studies

Case 1: 13 year-old girl with fatigue, learning difficulty, allergies

Diagnosis
Undiagnosed

Presenting symptoms
Extreme fatigue
Eczema
Patches of inflamed skin, behind knees, elbows, undiagnosed
Learning difficulty, visual dyslexia, with difficulty reading and remembering
Hay fever.

Medical history
Spontaneous ear drum perforation at ages 2, 3 5 and 7
"Asthma" age 4. *Intal* used without success, then used *Flixotide* as needed.
Easy bruising, even as a toddler. Skin splits and won't heal.
Hyper-mobile joints – dislocation of right elbow 20 times!
Ongoing fatigue, poor sleep patterns, difficult concentration and memory
Long history of undiagnosed abdominal pain
Uncoordinated and slow walking as a toddler.

Investigations
Gliadin antibodies – negative
Red Blood Cells and Haemoglobin - normal
Epstein Barr virus – past exposure (IgG positive)
Sleep study – no sleep apnoea detected.

Current medications
Flixotide
Zyrtec
Dermaid
Various naturopathic supplements: Omega-3, immune herbs, acidophilus, zinc

General impression
- An intelligent, quiet child, always tired, and always suffering from something – eczema, skin lesions, fatigue. She wakes tired, despite 11 hours sleep (sometimes restless) and normal red cells and iron.
- 3-4 nights of the week she has nightmares
- Dark circles under the eyes with lymphatic congestion
- She has very tight facial skin, with wrinkles remaining after I pull down her lower lids
- Long history of umbilical pain (undiagnosed) after meals.

Particulars
- Lip splitting
- Food triggers: colourings, preservatives.

Generals
- Cold sensitive+++

Assessment
I first thought about the underpinning cause.
- On the symptoms alone there is likely to be heavy metal toxicity. Having requested a HTMA for this patient to verify this and assess the amount in the tissue, I move on to the second issue:
- Possible chronic intestinal parasitosis. The following symptoms suggest this: umbilical pain; restless sleep; night terrors. I decide to start treatment here as the first layer of the chronic disease, whose symptoms make a strong presence.
- There may also be a deficiency of magnesium and calcium, given the difficulty with sleep. The HTMA will confirm this. In the meantime I assume a deficiency and prescribe those minerals as supplements to help with sleep.

First Prescription
- *Cina 200c*: one dose every second day until the next visit
- Calcium and magnesium supplement at bedtime to aid restful sleep.

First Follow up[123]
- Sleep quality > (she is less restless)
- No skin flare ups
- No night terrors
- No tummy pain

Comments and Second Treatment
- Improvement. Chronic parasitic infection was likely, now cleared by *Cina*.
- HTMA shows cadmium toxicity, as suspected. I now know that a deeper layer of the pathology is the accumulation of this toxic element.
- *CH77*[124]: 3 mls daily. This is a gentle, general chelation agent, as described in Chapter 4.
- *Spatone* (iron supplement – conjunctiva are pale in spite of normal red cells and haemoglobin))

---

[123] Follow ups are usually every six weeks
[124] www.harmonology.com.au

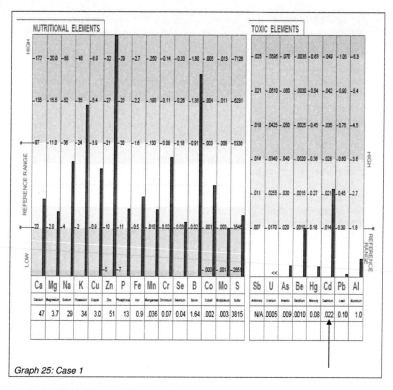

Graph 25: Case 1

Second Follow up and Treatment
- Fatigue 50% >
- Concentration >
- Some skin flare ups, but faster recovery
- A few colds, but fast recovery
- 'She's the best she's been for a long time'
- Continue CH77 & Spatone.

Third Follow up and Treatment
- Further improvement fatigue and concentration
- Skin > no itch; fewer flare ups; less severe
- Less cold sensitive (generals improve)
- Sleep much calmer – no nightmares
- Happier, not so grumpy (generals improve)
- Concentration >
- No abdominal pain
- Lip splitting continues

125

- Continue treatment. Add selenium 2 drops daily and iron supplement. Rationale: selenium is an immune stimulant and will help to remove the cadmium.

Fourth Follow up
- Top scoring in her history exams – doing very well with concentration and energy levels
- Wakes refreshed
- All other symptoms >
- New symptom: pins and needles in either foot, up to her thigh, most days, when sitting, lasting a few minutes
- New symptom: itching scalp with dry, flaking
- She is well, despite two new symptoms, so I continue same treatment.

Fifth Follow up
- All symptoms continue to improve
- The new symptoms (pins and needles and itchy scalp) have cleared up
- Continue same treatment

Sixth Follow up
- All symptoms further improved.
- Tried some trigger foods eg strawberries, without experiencing the usual skin aggravations.
- Today she has a staphylococcal skin infection with itching and yellow discharge, for which she normally takes antibiotics.
- We discuss a non-antibiotic treatment option: *Arsenicum 200c + Staph aureus 12c*
- Continue same treatment protocol.

Seventh Follow up
- Aggravation of skin after last visit; antibiotics given.
- Following this the patient caught a "virus" with fever, headache, dizziness, for three days.
- After this, she is symptom free, including no food triggers, no asthma. It seems like the "virus" was an aggravation from the homeopathic remedies, taking into account this girl's subsequent improvement.
- The next HTMA shows that the cadmium is only being excreted slowly (the first Cadmium reading was .022mg%; the follow up was 0.17mg%). Consequently I give a more specific chelation treatment: *Cadmium Chelate*: one dose every second day for eight weeks. Other toxic elements have been well excreted. This highlights the constitutional issue with this patient: she has a very poor ability to excrete cadmium, even with a general chelation therapy. It is therefore more appropriate to prescribe the *Cadmium Chelate*, since this will:
- More rapidly excrete the cadmium
- Alter the patient's constitutional susceptibility to cadmium accumulation.

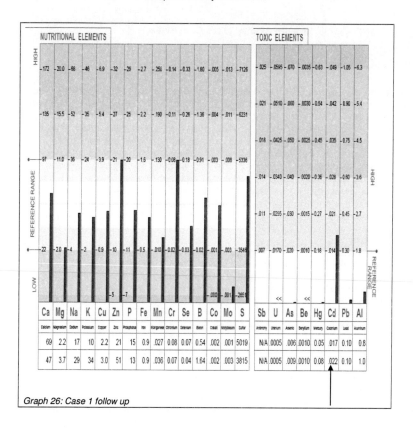

Graph 26: Case 1 follow up

Eight Follow up

The patient is symptom free. She enjoys good health and is discharged.

At 12 month follow up, she has been well.

Case 2: Boy of 14 with 'Allergy to his Own Sweat'

Diagnosis
'Non-specific atopy'

I first saw this boy at the age of 12 with allergic symptoms which occurred after exercise. He described this as 'I'm allergic to my own sweat'. He described a dry, sore throat accompanied by dyspnoea, a feeling of heat, prickling and swelling about the eyes and a skin rash. Initially both eyes had been affected but had recently localised to the right eye. The symptoms were aggravated by physical activity and hot weather. There was a history of severe asthma at 7 months of age and a family history of hay fever and asthma. In general, the patient reported moderate energy levels and a desire for spicy foods. He suffered from sinus problems, snoring and mouth breathing and found that he slept better on his front, although he still woke up feeling tired.

Treatment
I prescribed remedies which appeared to be effective at the time, namely *Hepar sulph 200c; Rhus tox 30c* and a mix of *Apis 6c + Histaminum 30c + Arsenicum 6c* to be used when he had the acute allergic symptoms. Later I gave him higher potencies of *Histaminum (50M)* and tried a 'constitutional remedy' *Phosphorus 30c.*

The treatment was (apparently) successful and this patient was largely free of symptoms for the next six years, after which he returned, feeling anxious about his condition. Here were his current symptoms:

Presenting Symptoms
- Headaches with neck pain
- Tingling down his arms and legs with vesiculation ('as though insects crawling in my muscles')
- Muscle pain in legs, arms and back
- Breathlessness
- Sinus symptoms: blocked nose, itchy throat (ie respiratory allergic symptoms reminiscent of his allergic symptoms four years earlier)
- Dizziness
- Occasional anxiety attacks.

These symptoms began in September 2008 during exam stress. It was now June 2009 and he had been to many practitioners, both allopathic and complementary, without improvement. Investigations had included MRI scan, lumbar puncture, various ultrasounds and blood tests. This helps to explain why he felt anxious.

Assessment
What are we treating? Five years later, heavy metal toxicity was now firmly on my radar screen. Previously, I gave remedies based on the symptom picture,

but this did not take into account the *cause* or the obstacle to cure. This new symptom picture suggested toxicity, so I tested the urine for heavy metals and referred for HTMA. The *TESSOL*[125] urinalysis showed immediate strong reddish-brown, consistent with the HTMA result which was received two weeks later:

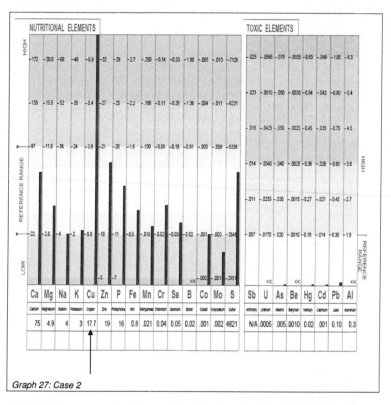

Graph 27: Case 2

This is a clear case of copper toxicity. The homeopathic treatment five years earlier, although 'successful', did not remove the cause of the disease. Similarly, if I had only repeated the prescriptions of five years earlier, there may again have been good improvement, but that treatment would not remove the copper toxicity, and he would relapse *with worse* symptoms again some time later. The homeopathic remedies, while effective in relieving his symptoms then, did not address this underlying toxicity, which requires a specific anti-*miasmatic* treatment. Without doing so the copper forms an obstacle to cure.

---

[125] www.harmonology.com.au

High copper is the most common metal toxicity I see in practice. Owing to the excessively high amount of copper coupled with the severe symptom presentation, I gave a double treatment protocol:

First Prescription
Copper chelate: one dose every second day plus the alkalising chelation agent *CH77*[126], 75 drops in a litre of water daily. In addition 30 mg elemental zinc tablet daily (since zinc is a copper antagonist).

First Follow up
This patient experienced good improvement in all symptoms at his first follow up four weeks later, with one small allergy attack after having a number of alcoholic drinks. Since copper is largely excreted through the liver, if the liver is challenged with other toxicities during the excretion process, then it is likely to bring on symptoms, as in this case.

While taking the *Copper Chelate* he was symptom free, yet after alcohol or becoming over tired his symptoms would start to recur. What is the assessment? First, his copper excretion was very slow on this treatment. Second, he is constitutionally very susceptible to the toxic effects of copper and will require a homeopathic remedy based on his symptom picture. Essentially, when his symptoms recur he experiences:
- Fatigue
- Restlessness
- Tingling or twitching in his muscles.

I prescribe *Zincum met 30c*: one dose every second day. Along with his zinc supplement and the *Copper Chelate*, this resolves his symptoms.

---

[126] CH77 is an oral chelation liquid containing low potency alkalising minerals

Case 3: Woman, age 40, with "foggy head", anxiety and insomnia

Diagnosis
unknown

Some cases require a mixture of constitutional prescribing combined with specific heavy metal detoxification using the methods described in Chapter 5. This is one such case, which shows us that the most rapid result of heavy metal removal is achieved with combination treatment plan.

I have given each consultation prescription in full so that the reader can see how the remedy choices were shaped by the changing presenting symptoms patterns. This patient's load of lead, initially 10 times off the graph, the largest load I have ever seen, was removed entirely in two months of specific chelation treatment. I would normally expect at least 12 months would be needed. A combination of constitutional prescribing and specific metal chelation gives the most efficient result.

Presenting symptoms
- Anxiety/hyper-vigilance < after day nap or night
- Fatigue
- Inability to think clearly or remember
- Insomnia.

General impression
- This single mother of two had a history of sexual abuse from age 6 to 10. She has always felt estranged. Her ex-husband did, and still does, play mind games with her, trying to control her. She suspects he is setting up their children for sexual abuse. She has anxiety at night, fearing her own death and imagining her children alone.
- She suffered from post-*Epstein Barr* Chronic Fatigue Syndrome ten years earlier. She "couldn't speak, move or eat for two years".
- My impression is that she is frozen in anxiety and sadness. She feels there is something wrong with her; that she is incapable of having a loving relationship. She does not have a sense of who she is. She is holding it all in tightly.
- "My stress is too high. I'm stuck in sadness when I stop. My brain doesn't work properly. I've improved my diet and am seeing a counsellor. There's something wrong with me. My mother hated me. I could never please her."
- "I go to speak, then I can't recall. I'm running and never stopping. I can't do enough to make my kids safe. Yet in all this I can never cry."
- "I am scared being alone. I panic on going to bed or waking after a day nap. I feel constant dread."
- "Recalling myself as a small girl it is black, dark, I am lost and alone."

Assessment
- This case has strong Chronic Fatigue Syndrome symptoms, and there has been a history of that syndrome.

- There is a long history of sexual abuse as a child.
- When she thinks of several key events in her life she experiences anxiety.
- This is a multi-layered case which will benefit from psychotherapy concurrently with homeopathic treatment. What are all those layers? We do not yet know, so I start treatment with the most striking symptom presentation, which is her anxiety:

First Prescription
Her first layer is anxiety / trauma / fear of the memory of her trauma; so I prescribe *Opium 30c*.

First Follow up *(follow ups are every 6 weeks unless otherwise stated)*
Anxiety was better until she and her children were witness to a truck accident. They were sitting in a restaurant when a truck lost its breaks and crashed through the window. They were not physically injured, but her anxiety has again increased. She pictures her children growing up without her.

Second Prescription
Opium 200c

Second Follow up
- Sleep >
- Hyper-vigilance >
- worrying less
- Ability to focus >
- Eating / appetite >
- No improvement to fatigue or memory.

Third Prescription
Opium 200c and Coxsackievirus 30c: one dose on alternate days. *Coxsackie* is added to the prescription because of the strong post-viral history. I use this nosode in the treatment of post-viral syndromes, especially post-Epstein Barr virus. She is starting to move into the *second layer* of the treatment.

Third Follow Up
- *Coxsackie* produced sore glands and pain in rib margins (old symptom). These were transient symptoms.[127]
- Anxiety and sleep quality > Waking each night around 1.00 but falling asleep again; no anxiety attacks.
- No significant change to fatigue or foggy head.

Fourth Prescription
Gelsemium 200c

---

[127] I have observed this symptom in several other patients with post-viral fatigue

132

Fourth Follow up *(9 months gap)*
- Exhaustion
- Sleep disturbed by overwhelming sadness
- Feeling safer, much less anxious
- Feels alone, lost, in the dark...."I'm dropping down a dark hole..."
- Foggy head has improved *slightly* on gels.
- Assessment: now the third layer – grief – is arising.

Fifth Prescription
Diamond Immersion 200c: one dose every second day.

Fifth Follow up
- "Best sleep in years after the remedy."
- Then some relapse. "Although sleep hours are better I am not getting the benefit, still waking tired. I feel like my body is fighting the remedy".
- "I feel alone when with friends."
- No change to fatigue, memory or foggy head.

Sixth Prescription
Diamond Immersion 1M[128], take as needed.

Sixth Follow Up
Sleep >
"I'm aware of something arising but I'm still running away from it."
Fatigue, memory and foggy head no >
TESSOL[129] test (urine) shows quick strong red. Referral for HTMA (below). Her lead level is *ten times* off the graph.

---

[128] A remedy proved by Peter Tumminello: *Twelve Jewels,* The Medicine Way, Sydney, 2005
[129] www.harmonology.com.au

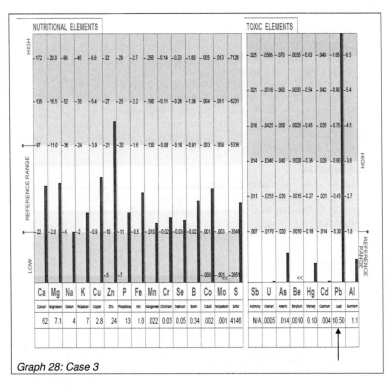

Graph 28: Case 3

Assessment

I now have a clearer picture of what I am treating. The uppermost layers of this disease matrix consist of anxiety and depression, which are clearly derived from life experience. In the next layer I can see a post-viral influence, which was the precipitating factor in her Chronic Fatigue Syndrome many years earlier. Now the HTMA shows the underlying lead toxicity which must is the cause of her foggy head and fatigue. Unless I remove it there will be an enduring obstacle to cure. Incidentally, it is the highest level I have seen. It is a very severe toxicity and explains many of the patient's enduring symptoms. It may explain why she 'could not move for two years' during her Chronic Fatigue Syndrome.

Her disease layers might look something like this:

Anxiety
Depression
Post-viral CFS
Heavy metal toxicity: lead

134

Seventh Prescription
CH77[130] 10 then up to 150 drops daily
Selenium 3 drops daily
Plumbum chelate one dose every second day
Iron supplement .

Seventh Follow Up
- Memory shows great improvement (at last!)
- Foggy head persists
- Sleep is OK as long as she keeps taking *Diamond*, however she is having ongoing battles with her ex-husband, causing her stress and disturbed sleep.
- "Hopeless, I can't see things getting any better. Yet stepping out of the fog is daunting"
- My impression is that the "fog" may cocoon her from her terror. It may have served her in this respect, in that she has been able to keep functioning as a single mother, despite her trauma. Had the full impact of her trauma been truly experienced, she may have not been able to keep functioning at all.

Eighth Prescription
Cimicifuga 30c: one dose every second day.

Eight Follow Up
- Fatigue much >
- Sleep "amazing"
- Depression < for 1st 10 days, then better.
- No anxiety!
- Foggy head much better
- Today she shows her *anger* for the first time when discussing what has happened in her life. She is now animated, and has breathed some life into her life story. This is a great therapeutic sign.
- Her foggy head is better, now she can read, enjoy it and retain it. She has started journaling and finds this beneficial.
- *TESSOL urine test* – green – despite such a high lead load. This means her lead has gone! She has been able to rapidly chelate the lead. Given the level of her load of the heavy metal lead, it is surprising, if not wonderful, that it has been excreted so quickly without any side effects. The combination of heavy metal chelation with constitutional treatment gave the most rapid result.

Ninth Prescription
Cimicifuga 200c: one dose every second day.

---

[130] CH77 is an oral chelation liquid containing low potency alkalising minerals

Ninth Follow Up
- Foggy head, memory, fatigue >>
- Night terror has returned:
- "Terror of something happening to me and kids are alone"
  - o Fearful thoughts at night
  - o Nothing is safe
  - o Not fitting in

Tenth Prescription
Stramonium 1M as needed. Use *Coffea 200c* for sleep as needed.

Tenth Follow Up
- *Coffea* was great for sleep. *Stramonium* significantly reduced her anxiety
- Symptom free. She feels well, with great sleep and energy. Patient is discharged.
- There is no relapse at her 12-month follow up.

Case 4, Four year-old girl

Presenting symptoms
- Loose stools with umbilical pain
- Offensive flatulence
- Recurring urinary tract infections
- Hyperactivity, sometimes with unexpected angry behaviour
- Disturbed sleep sometimes with nightmares
- History of colic and poor digestion.

Observation
- White spots on fingernails
- Restless, all over the room during the consultation.

What are we treating?
- Chronic intestinal parasites, evidenced by umbilical pain, disturbed sleep, angry behaviour, smelly flatulence
- HTMA shows a huge toxic load of mercury, cadmium and copper.
- High mercury or copper loads provide a fertile environment for chronic parasitosis.

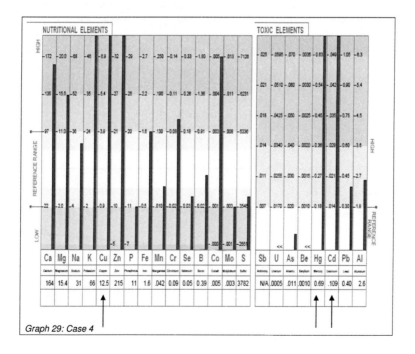

Graph 29: Case 4

Treatment Summary
- A long course of *Cina 200c*, one dose every second day for several months. This was followed by a course of *Stannum 200c*, specific for parasitic generated umbilical pain, also for several months. This improved the digestive symptoms, especially the abdominal pain, loose stools, smelly wind, and some improvement in sleep quality and angry behaviour.
- Concurrently with the above treatment, I prescribed an alkalising chelation agent, *CH77*[131], 30 to 40 drops daily in water, for 12 months. This child has salivary tissue pH of 7.0 which is ideal tissue alkalinity for natural chelation of toxic elements. I used *CH77*, rather than a single homeopathic metal chelator, because of the cocktail of toxic elements present. I do not know which is any of them is involved in her symptoms, and I want her to gently excrete all those elements.

Outcome
The patient was well after 12 months of treatment for intestinal parasites and a surprisingly high toxic load. The same load was also found in her sister. Her father also had these toxic elements, though much less.

I was unsure as to whether there was an exogenous exposure with this family, since the family history did not reveal a possible source. It is likely that cases like this have a genetic or constitutional propensity to retain toxic elements, even though the patient is comparatively well in spite of the large toxic load. If a similar toxic element pattern is found in siblings and parents, this indicates either a genetic or constitutional problem with toxic excretion or an external source.

---

[131] www.harmonology.com.au

Case 5: 14 year-old male

Diagnosis
Meniere's Disease, headaches, epilepsy

Presenting Symptoms
- Dizziness
- Vomiting
- Always tired
- Headaches
- Recurring "attacks" of dizziness and fainting at which time:
  o Unable to stand – faints
  o Facial pallor
  o Flushed face
  o Looks intoxicated
- Restless sleep
- Tinnitus with reduced hearing
- Tremor.

Other symptoms & History
Mild functional epilepsy (*petit mal*) with fainting and fevers as a child.
Taking *Tegratol* for some years then.
Sleepwalking, fainting and vomiting.
Eyes roll backward during these fits.

Generals
Very chilly

Assessment
Meniere's disease with prior history of petit mal epilepsy for which he had been given *Tegretol* (not currently). However, the symptom picture suggested the petit mal was still active.

First Prescription
- *China sulph 30c* : one dose every second day
- *Belladonna 200c*: take only as needed for acute attacks of dizziness and fainting
- Zinc supplement (he has white spots on his fingernails).

First follow up
- *Belladonna* was effective for reducing frequency and severity of the attacks
- No change to tinnitus, though slight improvement in hearing
- Urine *TESSOL*[132] test suggested a high level of copper, which is neurotoxic.

---

[132] An instant heavy metal test of the patient's urine: www.harmonology.com.au

Second prescription
- Continue first prescription
- Add: *CH77*[133], 75 drops daily. Presuming there is a copper toxicity, I add some gentle chelation drops.

Second follow up
- Fewer attacks, less duration and intensity, with *Belladonna* being used successfully when needed.
- No further change to tinnitus or deafness. For this reason I ordered a HTMA, which revealed a high level of copper, as suspected. The graph below shows before (14.1) and after three months of treatment (9.2) with a steady decrease in the copper level.

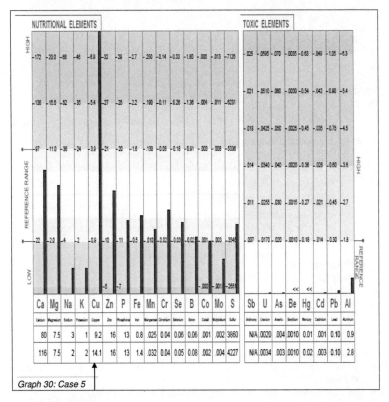

Ca	Mg	Na	K	Cu	Zn	P	Fe	Mn	Cr	Se	B	Co	Mo	S	Sb	U	As	Be	Hg	Cd	Pb	Al
Calcium	Magnesium	Sodium	Potassium	Copper	Zinc	Phosphorus	Iron	Manganese	Chromium	Selenium	Boron	Cobalt	Molybdenum	Sulfur	Antimony	Uranium	Arsenic	Beryllium	Mercury	Cadmium	Lead	Aluminum
80	7.5	3	1	9.2	16	13	0.8	.025	0.04	0.06	0.06	.001	.002	3860	N/A	.0020	.004	.0010	0.01	.001	0.10	0.9
116	7.5	2	2	14.1	16	13	1.4	.032	0.04	0.05	0.08	.002	.004	4227	N/A	.0034	.003	.0010	0.02	.003	0.10	2.8

Graph 30: Case 5

Third prescription
Continue above
Add *Copper chelate* – one dose every second day.

---

[133] CH77 is an oral chelation liquid containing low potency alkalising minerals

Third follow up
- No attacks since last visit.
- No dizziness
- No vomiting
- NO TINNITUS
- No tremor
- Now wearing hearing aid

It is clear from this case that copper toxicity underpinned the patient's 'epilepsy' and the Meniere's disease.

Case 6: 9 year- old boy

Diagnosis
Asperger's syndrome; Attention Deficit Hyperactivity Disorder

This nine year old boy displayed aggressive, unco-operative and sometimes antisocial behaviour. He did not make friends easily; his interest was more on reading books (he was ahead of his years in reading skills) and computers (he sneaks into the home office to use the computer). He suffered from fluctuations in energy – either hyperactive or fatigued. When under stress, as he often was at school, he would run away. He was defiant, unco-operative, frequently interrupted the conversation I was having in clinic with his mother. He was very curious, interested in space, animals and science, and asked lots of questions.

> He was focussed on gun and wars: "I want to shoot you". His dreams are full of aliens killing people.
> He speaks in a loud voice, often shouting.
> He must be the centre of attention; he "depletes everyone's energy".
> He is too rough when playing with other children. When he is angry he is very strong.

He had a strong craving for sweets. Sometimes he would get up in the middle of the night and sneak into the kitchen to seek out sweet foods. It also took him a long time to fall asleep.

- He is a messy child.
- He suffered from chronic nose block and consequently was a mouth breather.
- At the time of consultation he was medicated with *Ritalin*.
- He was a very hot, sweaty child.
- There was a family history of depression and drug use.

The HTMA below is typical of children diagnosed with ADHD. Very high copper, almost four times off the chart, has to be removed for cure to take place. Constitutionally, this was a *sulphur* child. I prescribed these remedies:

- *Copper chelate* – one dose once every second day
- *Sulphur 6c* – one dose on each alternate day.
- Zinc
- Selenium.

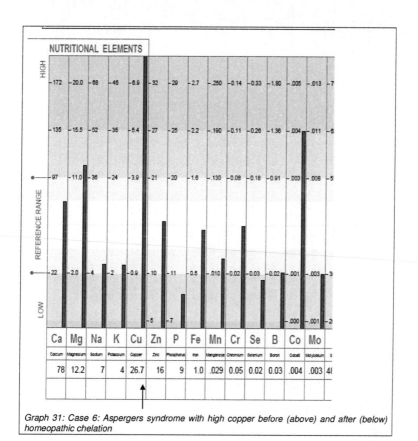

Graph 31: Case 6: Aspergers syndrome with high copper before (above) and after (below) homeopathic chelation

Over the ensuing nine months, this boy did very well in all the major symptoms:

Peaceful, calm sleep, no nightmares or waking

Calmer, better focussed, more able to be reasoned with

Able to stay on task much better

Better person to person contact; he begins making good eye contact

Aggression and tantrums much better

Anxiety is better

He Is "not so intense" – everyone can relax around him

Sweet cravings are much reduced

Nose cleared after many years of blockage.

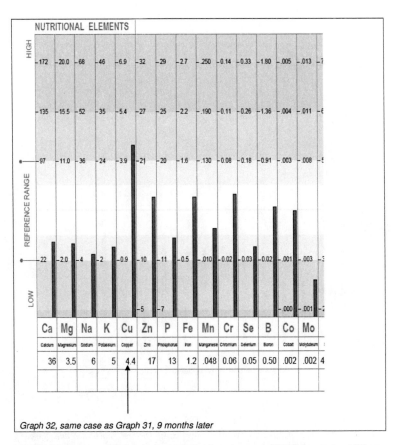

Graph 32, same case as Graph 31, 9 months later

Copper toxicity underpins hyperactivity disorder and ADHD in many children and is easily removed by using *Copper chelate* in conjunction with the constitutional remedy. His follow up HTMA, taken nine months later, shows the effectiveness of homeopathic chelation on copper:

144

Chapter 10
Toxic Chemical Case Studies

Case 7, male 46

Diagnosis
Squamous Cell Carcinoma with multiple secondaries

This man, an electrician, was a robust, jovial patient whom I had met some years earlier when his then partner was diagnosed with end stage cancer. Subsequent treatments for himself centred around blood pressure and stress management. He was a heavy smoker. Eventually a squamous cell carcinoma was found on his scalp, hidden beneath a healthy crop of hair. When it was discovered, it had already metastasised into his brain and down through his spinal column into his rib cage. In the words of his oncologist, his ribcage looked like "swiss cheese".

The patient decided to take homeopathic treatment concurrently with his chemotherapy, especially considering his prognosis was grim.

Over the next two years I used an alternating regime of *Arsenicum album*, starting at 200c and increasing to 50M; and *Carcinosin*, in the same potencies. I used the method advocated by Dr Ramakrishnan, giving frequent, plussed doses of the remedies.[134]

In addition, I give these supplements to all patients with cancer:
- Selenium – dose varies depending on type of cancer and the patient's nutritional status of selenium
- 'Liquid Oxygen' (liquid electrolytes of oxygen) – 50 drops daily
- Daily juicing with beetroot and carrot.

I continued this treatment for two years, during which time there was no evidence of continued cancer activity. The patient was in good health except for ongoing deep bone pain in his spine and ribcage. I then gave a concurrent treatment to heal the bone lesions: *Symphytum 200c:* one dose every 2nd day plus *Calcarea phos 4x:* two doses daily.

After six months on this protocol the oncologist could not believe that the bony lesions had disappeared. The patient was completely free of bone pain.

I kept the patient on a maintenance dose of the *Arsenicum* and *Carcinosin*. Although in good health, *every month* he developed new skin cancers and had to have them either excised or burned off. Some of these were thought to be basal cell carcinomas, not as serious as the squamous cells, but nonetheless this showed there was still a primary carcinogenic causation manifesting on the patient's skin.

---

[134] Ramakrishnan, Dr A, *A Homeopathic Approach to Cancer,* Quality Medical Publishing Inc, Missouri, 2001

Further questioning of the patient revealed that he had grown his own vegetables for over 20 years, and here is the list of pesticides and herbicides he used:

1. **Tomato Dust** – Sulphur, Copper Oxychloride & Spinosad.
2. **Vegetable Dust** – Derris & Rotenone.
3. **Chemspray Mancozeb** – Mancozeb.
4. **Chemspray Zineb** – Zineb.
5. **Pyrethrum Insecticide** – Pyrethrins. & Pyperonyl.
6. **Diazinon** – used in 1993.
7. **Lawn & Grub Killer** – Chlorpyrifos.
8. **Bin-Die** – Bromoxynil, MCPA & Hydrocarbon Liquid.
9. **Baysol Snail & Slug** – Methiocarb.
10. **Lebaycid** – Fenthion.
11. **Zero** – Glyphosate.

I was shocked, but after my shock subsided, I realised this is not unusual It reminded me how people are unaware that the garden chemicals they use are so toxic. Just because they are, or were, legal, does not make them safe. Especially if you are eating them!

At one time, *Diazinon* and *Mancozeb* were legal pesticides you could buy at your local hardware store. Since they were declared carcinogenic they are now banned. All the while these were still in his garden shed, this patient had been continuing to use these chemicals in his vegetable garden. Was this was the primary toxicity underlying his cancer diathesis. *Diazinon* has been shown to increase the incidence of brain cancers.[135]

Accordingly I prescribed the *Pesticide, Herbicide & Fungicide Protocol*, which is described in Chapter 6:

Pesticide, Herbicide & Fungicide Protocol 200c: 3 doses on Day 1.
Pesticide, Herbicide & Fungicide Protocol 30c: 3 doses on Day 2.
Pesticide, Herbicide & Fungicide Protocol 16c: 3 doses on Day 3.
No medicine on Day 4.
Pesticide, Herbicide & Fungicide Protocol 16c: 3 doses on Day 5
Pesticide, Herbicide & Fungicide Protocol 30c: 3 doses on Day 6.
Pesticide, Herbicide & Fungicide Protocol 200c: 3 doses on Day 7.

After this protocol, the patient's skin cancers stopped, and he has been symptom free.

---

[135] Cox, Caroline, "Carbaryl," Journal of Pesticide Reform, Spring 1993:13(1), Northwest Coalition for Alternatives to Pesticides, Eugene, OR. http://panna.igc.org/resources/pestis/PESTIS.1996.18.html.

Chapter 11
Iatrogenic Case Studies

Vaccinosis

Case 8: four year-old boy

This boy was non-verbal at four years old. Many of his type of symptoms present in children diagnosed on the autistic spectrum: speech delay, refusal to make eye contact and dislike for being touched. He had not been diagnosed, but if his symptom picture failed to improve, 'autistic' would almost certainly have been his eventual diagnosis.

Presenting Symptoms
- Abdominal pain
- Head banging
- Hypersensitivity reactions to many foods.
- Irritable, cross, resists attempts by parents for affection. Doesn't want to be touched especially on the head, or looked at.
- Makes poor eye contact
- Night terrors.
- Non verbal – only made the sound 'buh'
- Offensive diarrhoea
- Ongoing headaches
- Poor appetite
- Pretends he's a dog and growls at people
- Temper tantrums for no obvious reason: Suddenly yells at strangers.

Food supplements
Neocate and Metameal.
He was placed on formula at birth, since his older brother had anaphylactic reactions to many foods.

History
- Birth: surgical repair of pyloric stenosis.
- 10 months: severe case of salmonella infection; hospitalised because of the severity of the diarrhoea.
- 11 months recurring ear infections, treated with antibiotics and grommets. His hearing became *worse* and then he *stopped talking.*

Family History
- Mother: adult onset allergies, anaphylaxis to nuts
- Mother's father: alcoholism and violence.

The most pressing problem was his chronic diarrhea and tummy pain: I chose to treat probable intestinal parasites first.

First prescription
Cina 200c one dose every second day.
Night terrors, abdominal pain and extreme irritability indicate parasitic infection.
During the next two weeks:
- Passed tiny black spots in his stools, which then became properly formed, and flatulence improved
- Appetite and abdominal pain improved slightly.
- Night terrors improved.

Despite these encouraging signs, there were minimal changes to his overall behavioural problems. Abdominal pain and headaches continued.

Second prescription
Nux vomica 30c alternating with *Stannum met 200c.*
- Fewer night terrors
- Less abdominal pain and flatulence.
- Still complained of infrequent headaches and abdominal pain.

I needed to take a 'layered' approach to treatment.

Suspect *vaccinosis* when you see symptoms like these:
- Symptoms beginning soon after vaccination
- Frequent waking
- Head-banging: without any evidence of middle ear infection, this is a sign of cerebral irritation, and can be a strong pointer to *vaccinosis.*
- Nocturnal fevers
- Ongoing unexplained coughs, colds, wheezing
- Repeated otitis media &/or middle ear effusion.
- Weight loss, poor appetite, picky eater

Third prescription:
DPT/Pedvax 30c, then 200c and finally 1M (in ascending order) one potency given each day after Dr Tinus Smit's protocol. [136]

The response to this prescription was incredible. One day he was an angry child who refused all affection. The next day he went to his mother and said for the first time: "I love you Mummy".
Over the next few weeks his speech development rocketed. His unexplained tantrums improved. The head banging stopped. His appetite improved. His bowel function completely returned to normal.

Rationale:
If I look at this patient in a layered approach, this is how I think his health was affected:

---

[136] http://www.post-vaccination-syndrome.com/3890/treatment.aspx

1. Mother had strong tendency to food allergy (with anaphylaxis). Possibly there are other genetic factors with the mother's father.
2. Child is born with this inherited tendency.
3. Child is given the usual vaccinations to which he reacts.
4. He contracts 'salmonella'
5. He has ongoing health problems affecting intestinal and nervous systems.

Treatment aimed to peel off these disease layers in *reverse* order:
1. Remove any intestinal pathogens
2. Antidote presumed side effects of vaccination
3. Constitutional or miasmatic prescription to reduce allergic and hypersensitive tendencies.

Fourth prescription:
A single dose of *Tuberculinum bov 10M*, provoked a high fever and sore throat. His writing skills began to develop. Tantrums were better, but he could still be violent with his brothers (biting, punching).

Now that so much of his disease pathology had been 'peeled off', I had the opportunity to observe his behaviour more clearly. The violent outbursts tended to occur whenever any attention was given to his brothers. In other words, he was jealous. There is a great little rubric in Peter Tumminello's repertory, *The Child's Mind and Behaviour*.[137] "Jealously, baby, when a new, takes the attention of the family away". We also find the rubric "Jealousy, rage, with" in Murphy's *Repertory*[138] with only one remedy.

Fifth prescription:
Hyoscyamus 1M, one dose. Since this remedy, behaviour has been excellent, with far fewer tantrums. His speech and writing are now excellent, and his speech is clear.

Cases like this, with a clinically indisputable result, confirm the view that vaccination can be a causative factor in *subsequent* disease. Otherwise, an antidote to that vaccine is unlikely to have had any effect. While a majority of children probably pass through the vaccination schedule without long-term side effects, there is a minority who do not. Certainly, in children with a strong family history of allergy or food sensitivity, the risk of vaccination needs to be carefully reviewed.

Swine Flu *Vaccinosis*
These two patients presented with chronic coughs.

- A woman of 58 presented with lymphoedema of the left arm which had

---

[137] Tumminello, P, *The Child's Mind and Behaviour,* The Medicine Way, Sydney, 2001
[138] Murphy, R, *Homeopathic Medical Repertory,* Hahnemann Academy of North America, 1993

followed an undiagnosed rash on that arm eight weeks earlier. She next developed yellow nasal mucus, a chronic wheeze and cough. A provisional diagnosis from her respiratory specialist was pulmonary sardoidosis. Her symptoms responded only minimally to *Augmentin* and *Ventolin*. I tried both *Kali carb 200c* and *Bryonia 30c,* which improved the cough and wheeze by 40 per cent after 3 weeks, with no further improvement. Further questioning revealed that the original symptoms appeared two days after her Swine Flu vaccination. Accordingly I prescribed three doses of *Swine Flu Nosode 200c,* after which all symptoms disappeared.

- In the second case, a 2½ year old girl came in with a constant early morning cough, worse at 4am, and wheezing, for the past 6 months. She had received a Swine Flu vaccination before starting day care, at 18 months of age. Her cough began two days after this vaccination. Three doses of *Swine Flu Nosode 200c* were given, which cleared the symptoms entirely.

Oral Contraceptive Pill

Case 9: 32 year-old woman
Some allopathic medications can leave an imprint on the nervous system, resulting in functional disturbance as they did with this 32-year-old woman.

Presenting symptoms
- Ongoing painful sinusitis
- Vaginal thrush
- Ongoing fatigue
- Aching
- Tingling in extremities.

History
She describes how she felt sick when on the oral contraceptive pill (OCP) many years earlier.
After the OCP, she had a contraceptive implant, which also made her feel sick and it caused a thrombosis.

Years later (when seeing me) she described her contraceptives medicines as the beginning of her health problems. The OCP essentially caused what became a chronic fatigue, with the aching, tiredness and tingling.

Prescription
Folliculinum 30c, one dose every second day for several weeks completely cleared her sinusitis and thrush.

When women have side effects during or when started the OCP, strongly consider this as an obstacle to cure. Women who have side effects often describe either headaches or mood disturbance since they started the OCP.

Antibiotics

The iatrogenic effects of antibiotics are often seen in practice. It is becoming more common for pregnant women to be given routine antibiotics just before delivery, especially if they tested positive for *Steptococcus B*. This brings the newborn child into the world already exposed to antibiotics, resulting in a degradation of the quality of the gut flora. Many newborn babies suffer terrible colic and food sensitivity as a result of this degradation of gut flora. Giving potentised antibiotics can improve this situation. However, in many cases the gut flora also requires restoration.[139] This situation, not uncommon, is especially unfortunate since giving homeopathic *Streptococcinum* to the mother for several days prior to the birth will almost certainly clear the evidence of Streptococcus from the blood test.

Children who receive antibiotics within their first six months of birth greatly increase their risk of developing allergies before the age of seven.[140]

Case 10: 7 month old baby girl – never well since antibiotics through breast milk

When a course of antibiotics had been prescribed to this breastfeeding mother for mastitis, it created a profound gut disturbance in her one week-old baby. The mother tried to treat her mastitis herself, without success. As soon as she started taking the antibiotics, her baby had developed projectile vomiting, severe colic, with abdominal pain being worse at night and disrupting her sleep. The baby then lost her appetite, became constipated and stopped gaining weight. She also developed symptoms of intestinal candida and parasites. The mother had a history of chronic vaginal thrush, which is often evidence of gut dysbiosis. Another course of antibiotics would aggravate this.

Prescriptions

- The baby improved when given potentised A*moxicillin.*
- Projectile vomiting improved with *Aethusa cynapium 200c*
- Night colic was well managed with *Colocynthis 200c.*
- The baby and all the family (see below) required ongoing treatment for intestinal parasites using *Cina 200c.*
- Antibiotics were the catalyst for the symptoms developing and required antidoting with potentised *Amoxicillin.*

Antibiotics denude the beneficial gut flora in susceptible patients and more likely create gut dysbiosis in already weakened gut flora. This can lead to a susceptibility to intestinal parasites.

Case 11: 29 year-old woman with recurring colds and sinusitis

This 29 year old woman had fatigue and recurring colds which 'lasted for months' at a stretch. She had a history of using lots of antibiotics for colds and

---

[139] The issue of deteriorating gut flora is discussed in Gamble, J, *Mastering Homeopathy 2 The Treatment of Irritable Bowel Syndrome,* Karuna Publishing, 2006
[140] http://www.sciencedaily.com/releases/2003/10/031001064200.htm

sinus infections. She had multiple courses of antibiotics as a child for tonsillitis. (The proving of penicillin shows strong sinus symptoms and can be considered as a remedy especially where many courses of antibiotics have been taken.)

After *Amoxicillin 30c*, she developed swollen glands, fatigue and a vague fluey feeling. Her chronic sinus congestion then cleared, as did her fatigue. Her facial acne also improved.

Prednisone

Case 12: Sleepwalking in a 26 year-old woman

This case is an example of the profound, while obscure, effect that allopathic medications can have on a patient. The neurological and emotional symptoms were entirely caused by a 'drug *miasm*': *Prednisone*. While I would have been tempted to give potentised *Prednisone* in this case, it was not needed because the *simillimum* was able to remove the entire disease layer and demonstrate Hering's Law of Cure. It is satisfying when the *simillimum* clears the whole case, however cases like this often require a *tautopathic* prescription.

Presenting symptoms
This 26-year-old woman had sleepwalking and nightmares. The nightmares caused her to jump out of bed screaming and run down the corridor. She only wakes up when her husband runs after her and catches her. She bumps into walls or objects and sometimes runs out of the house. She is concerned about seriously injuring herself.

Two dreams recur and are what cause her to leap out of bed. In the first, a wardrobe is about to fall and crush her and she must scramble to avoid it. In the second, her baby is falling off the bed and she must quickly catch her before she falls off. Her eyes are open, yet she remains asleep, so it is sleepwalking. Despite this regular experience, she is a sound sleeper.

Mentals and Generals
- "I talk too much. I'm dominant and set in my ways. I thrive on company."
- Always moving. Can't be still.
- Anxiety for others
- Chilly
- Desires company
- Desires: salt (3), spicy, salami, cheese, ice cold drinks (3).
- Fastidious: everything must be in its right place
- Fear of ghosts
- Fears deep water
- Fears the supernatural and her own psychic ability: "I fear entering old buildings because I can pick up on things".
- Loves animals and is sympathetic
- Somnambulism.

History
- Crohn's Disease, confirmed by endoscopy and treated with prednisone. The disease is now dormant.
- Large adenoids as a child.
- Benign growth on vocal chords causing hoarseness and pain > cold drinks.
- Nose bleeds as a child.

I prescribed *Phosphorus 200c*, which rapidly cured the nightmares and sleepwalking. However, three months later there was a return of the abdominal pain, which she had experienced earlier with the Crohn's Disease. She had been in 'remission' from this disease for almost two years.

What are we treating?
The primary disease state, the Crohn's Disease, was suppressed (happily, for this patient) by the *Prednisone* which gave rise to a deeper 'pathology', of sleepwalking and nightmares. According to Hering's Law, mind disturbance is a more serious disease layer than gut symptoms.

This iatrogenic disease suppression formed an obstacle to cure. In this case, only the constitutional medicine was needed to address both the deeper disease layer caused by the suppression; and the original disease formation, that is, the Crohn's Disease.

This is a clear example of Hering's Law, with the re-appearance of an earlier disease with the disappearance of the more recent presenting symptoms, from 'above downwards and from within to without'.

No further medicine was needed, as the abdominal pain was a transient symptom. At 12 months follow up, neither the abdominal pain nor nightmares had returned. Only one dose of *Phosphorus* was needed.
.

Chapter 12
Infection Case Studies

Ongoing sub-clinical infection, or the effects of a past infection, is not always obvious in a patient's case. If the *simillimum* is ineffective, this is a possible obstacle to cure which calls for meticulous case taking. It also demands detailed recall from the patient.

Swine Flu
When treating patients who have an infection, particularly a viral infection, giving the *nosode* of that virus in addition to the *similimum,* generally yields a more rapid resolution of the illness. I have used this method for many years, but its relevance became very apparent when treating patients with H1N1 Swine Flu over the last two winters.

In 2009 I did not have the *Swine Flu Nosode*, so had to rely on traditional influenza remedies.

Presenting symptoms of Swine Flu were:
• Rapid onset
• Sudden weakness
• High fever (39-40 degrees)
• Sore throat
• Headache
• Painful, debilitating, deep chest cough
• Deep, hollow barking cough with weakness.

In 2009 I used *Phosphorus 10M* for most patients, initially every two hours. All patients reported continuous improvement over the next few days with complete resolution after one week, and fortunately none of them went on to the tertiary stage of the virus: pneumonia.

By 2010 I had acquired the *Swine Flu Nosode* and was able to use it as both prophylactic and treatment for Swine Flu, as the following obstinate case of Swine Flu demonstrates.

Case 13: Obstinate Swine Flu

After using 'pink batt' fiberglass in his home renovation, this 50-year-old male felt weak in the chest and shortly afterwards developed a short, dry, painful chest cough with fever. I prescribed *Bryonia 200c*. With little improvement, after five days the cough was focused more in his trachea, with a loud, barking cough, and so next I prescribed *Spongia 30c*. A few days later he returned with painful mouth ulcers, thick tongue coating and a sore throat, and I next gave him *Mercurius sol 200c*. Although feeling better, he relapsed with the original painful chest cough, body aches, headache, and debilitating weakness and malaise. He (and I) were worried by this stage. It was then that I realised he had **Swine Flu**: although no pathology was done, I recognised the cough and extreme debility, which I had seen in the previous year's influenza season. Accordingly I next gave the *Swine Flu Nosode 200c*, one dose daily, with *Lycopodium 10M*. I prescribed the latter because of the late afternoon aggravation and symptoms were worse on the right side. None was as surprised as I when the entire cough and influenza symptoms cleared completely within **24 hours**. It is as though the *nosode* directs the curative power of the homeopathic remedy directly into the disease state.

Recurring fevers always suggest an infection which has not been properly expelled by the body: this can include a host of microorganisms: bacterial, viral or parasitic.

Case 14: Infection and kidney scarring in a young boy

I first saw this boy when he was five years, and gave him treatment at various intervals over the next five years.

When he was a baby, this boy had undiagnosed kidney reflux; the only symptom was recurring fevers. By the time he was diagnosed there was significant kidney scarring. He had a surgical correction followed by annual ultrasound of the kidneys to monitor size and growth.

When I first saw him, he presented with the symptoms of headaches, poor appetite and growing pains for which I successfully gave *Calcarea Phos 30c* and an iron supplement. After this, I prescribed a 12-month course of *Berberis 200c,* one dose every second day, to repair the kidney damage. After a year there were no signs of kidney trouble, His renal specialist was satisfied, but now he had recurring bouts of tonsillitis, for which I gave several acute prescriptions: *Mercurius cy 200c; Hepar sulph 200c; Belladonna 200c.* Although he always responded well to these acute prescriptions, he never had normal levels of energy or enthusiasm for his age. Compared to his two brothers, he has always tired, complaining often of sore bones including the hips, swollen glands, occasional fevers and sore throats. While 'growing pains' commonly occur in children, the locations is not usually the hips. I gave the *Ross River Fever Nosode 30c,* which spiked a fever and then cleared all his symptoms for the next 10 months. Then the fevers returned: these were only nocturnal and reached up to 40 degrees Celsius but without the other symptoms. Taking into account the history of tonsillitis and before that, the long history of urinary tract infections, I gave the *nosode Streptococcus Viridans 15c,* once every second day for three weeks. This finally put an end to his fevers.

Streptococcus is a common causation for kidney infections and tonsillitis in young children. The specific nosode was required to expel the pathogenic *miasm.*

Case 15: 18-year-old female
This was one of those cases where it was difficult to pin down the patient to precise information. Her memory was poor and it was clear that keeping her concentration and clarity required a sustained effort.

Presenting symptoms (since 5 years of age)
- Fatigue
- Poor concentration. Hard to focus on anything. "Head is full of cotton wool"
- Dizzy head
- Headaches, daily, just above the eyes
- Sore joints; knees, wrists, hips, sometimes with swelling, redness and heat
- Swollen cervical glands
- Recurring 'flus' – aching muscles, heavy head, elevated temperature.
- Sleep – OK
- No cravings.

History
She reacted to *Triple Antigen* (DPT) vaccine at 6 months of age, with high fever and "stiffness in the hips and legs." What this means and how her mother was aware that her baby had stiffness after vaccination, was not clear.

In the following few years there were two more significant disease events:
- Bell's Palsy.
- Encephalitis with high fever: the causative pathogen was not known.

Whether these latter two disease events were related to the reaction to vaccination is unclear. There is though, an apparent predisposition to disturbances of the nervous system. Whether this predisposition is due to her vaccination reaction can only ever be a mute point.

First prescription:
On totality of symptoms including the "cotton wool" head, heavy headaches, dizziness, recurring flu-type symptoms and history of encephalopathy, I chose *Gelsemium 200c,* once every second day for four weeks.

Follow up
She improved well on *Gelsemium.* The recurring "flu" symptoms resolved. The headaches were better, yet still occurring regularly. Fatigue was much better. Swollen glands were better. However, there was no improvement to the joint pain.

I prescribed on the totality of symptoms did not ask *what is causing her symptoms?* I did not '*identify what is to be treated'.*[141]

As I have discovered, the *totality of symptoms* treatment approach is not always adequate in *isolation* if there is a causative agent of disease. It is an obstacle to cure.

---

[141] Organon S. Hahnemann Aphorisms 3-5

What are we treating? What is the differential diagnosis?

Chronic fatigue syndrome?
For a diagnosis of Chronic Fatigue Syndrome (CFS) to be made, the patient must have at least three of the following symptoms for several months:
- Extreme fatigue not improved by rest
- Post-exertion malaise
- Fibromyalgia
- Muscle weakness
- Impaired memory and concentration
- Insomnia
- Ongoing sore throat and tender lymph nodes
- Joint pain without inflammation
- Chronic headaches
- Dizziness.

The characteristic feature of CFS, which is unrefreshing sleep, was not present in this case. Nor does CFS have the inflamed joints experienced by this patient.

Fibromyalgia?
- Generalised muscle pain with at least 11 tender points distributed over all quadrants of the body
- Paraesthesia
- Skin sensitivity
- Temporomandibular joint syndrome.

There were no tender points. Fibromyalgia does not have joint inflammation; it is a *soft tissue* inflammatory disorder.

Rheumatoid Arthritis?
In Rheumatoid Arthritis (RA) there are red, inflamed joints in the acute phase, with deformity of the joints in the chronic stages. It tends to affect the body symmetrically and can occur in children. However, RA does not have cognitive symptoms, unexplained fatigue and headaches or swollen lymphatic glands.

Multiple Sclerosis?
Multiple sclerosis has:
- Fatigue
- Eye pain
- Spasticity
- Tremor
- Progressive loss of vision, sensation and motor control.

Apart from this patient's fatigue, none of these other symptoms are present.

Vaccinosis?
Homeopathically speaking, it is tempting to diagnose this girl's symptoms as arising from *vaccinosis* given her reaction to the 6 month of age *Triple Antigen*

vaccination, especially since pain and stiffness in her hip joints was one of the presenting although transient symptoms afterwards.

I have made these differential diagnoses in writing up this case, because it is useful to illustrate the point that: as practitioners we need to understand what we are treating. I think any homeopath would consider vaccinosis as possible disease causation. However, this girl's doctor had thought that a possible aetiology was *Lyme Disease* to which after a blood test, she tested positive. This was the first case of Lyme Disease that I had knowingly treated.

Accordingly, when I found out that my patient had *Lyme Disease,* I gave *Lyme Disease Nosode 10M,* one dose weekly, with advice to continue until no symptoms, or stop if there is a change or aggravation of symptoms.

I added this *nosode* because:
• I had no experience at this time of treating Lyme Disease, a bacterial infection, so was unsure whether *Gelsemium* would be palliative or curative
• Lyme Disease is a destructive disease and it had many years start on me to begin its work in this patient
• I felt an isopathic prescription or *nosode* would boost the effect of *Gelsemium.*

I did not hear from the patient for another two years, when I discovered that she had gone on to a full remission of all her symptoms! The use of the *Lyme Disease Nosode* and *Gelsemium* were instrumental in bringing about this remission. I am uncertain how many doses of the *nosode* my patient took, because of the two year gap, so the information by then was lost to history. I gather it was a prompt and steady response given that she felt no need to make contact again after the prescription.

I had never treated Lyme Disease before and the use of the *nosode* was a guess. But I got it right! I am not sure whether I would necessarily use *Gelsemium* again if I saw this case today.

The other surprising thing for me is that no further medicine was needed. Did the patient's history of reaction to vaccination and history of encephalitis create a fertile ground for seeds of a later Borrelia infection? A history of vaccinosis or encephalopathy is mentioned by Alex as predisposing factors to Lyme disease.

Even if I had prescribed *Gelsemium* on the basis of the totality of symptoms, the result may not have been as satisfactory. Peter Alex[142] says that this disease can easily be (and often is) misdiagnosed as any of the differential diagnoses mentioned above. Unless the specific blood test is done, *Lyme* can be a hidden disease, not dissimilar to the way syphilis (in the same,

---

[142] Alex, Peter, *The Homeopathic Treatment of Lyme Disease*, HomeopathyWest Publishing, 2006

spirochaete family) silently moves deeper through its three stages of manifestation also causing arthropathy and neurologic abnormalities. Consequently, Alex describes this disease as a '*Lyme miasm*' - an appropriate description given the hidden, latent nature of the illness.

Using *Lyme Disease Nosode* is a common practice in Europe for the treatment of Lyme disease.

Lyme Disease

Lyme Disease is a chronic disease caused by a bacterial (spirochaete) infection with *Borrelia bergdorferei*. (The syphilis organism, *Treponema Pallidum,* is also a spirochaete) It is transmitted by deer tick bite of the *Ixodes ricinus*. Lyme Disease was first named in the 1970s after there was an unusual number of cases of what appeared to be juvenile rheumatoid arthritis in the Old Lyme region of Connecticut, USA. Lyme Disease is prevalent in many countries throughout the world, especially Europe and North America, but also in parts of China, Russia and Japan. Although not officially acknowledged in Australia, cases present.

There are three distinct phases of manifestation:

Acute phase: following the tick bite, there is a bull's eye type rash soon after, or many weeks after, the initial bite which can last for a few weeks. The rash is called *erythema migrans*. The patient has usually forgotten about the bite by the time symptoms appear. As well as the rash there may be non-specific symptoms such as vague flu-like symptoms, fatigue and glandular swellings.

Secondary phase: later – and it may be many years later, the joint inflammatory stage begins. The patient is unlikely to make any connection between the joint pain and the old tick bite; particularly if there have been many previous tic bites. Some patients only develop vague symptoms of malaise and fatigue, so it is easy to confuse *Lyme Disease* with CFS, while other patients may go on to develop fibromyalgia.

Tertiary phase: the nervous system becomes involved, with cognition being affected. As in this case, there is difficulty in concentration. There may be memory loss or distorted or exaggerated sense reception. Other symptoms can be paralysis, vertigo or neuralgia. Cases of meningo-encephalitis, cranial neuritis (especially Bell's palsy) and motor radiculo-neuropathies have also been reported.

Here is another case of Lyme Disease, which I saw many years later:

Case 16: 45 year old man

Diagnosis: nil

Presenting Symptoms
- "There is a virus attacking my joints"
- There is joint pain in the wrists and ankles
- "It feels like a nail in my joints"
- My arms and legs feel like they have weights stretching them"
- Fatigue.

Aetiology
Four weeks prior to the consultation:
"It started after flu symptoms, after a stressful time at work."

Modalities
Better for rest and heat

Generals/Particulars
- Night sweats
- Headaches, dizziness.

History
- Teens: Undiagnosed joint pain in the hips and groin for a several weeks. Diagnosis was 'joint pain'.
- 35 years: hospitalised for a viral chest infection
- Two kidney stone procedures (lithotripsy).

Unlike the previous case, the disease was detected in its early stage by blood test and the symptom picture was focused mainly in the musculo-skeletal system.

Prescription
- *Rhus tox 30c* starting three times daily, slowly reducing to one dose every second day.
- *Lyme Disease Nosode 30c*, following Alex's protocol, mentioned above.[143]

All symptoms had cleared after four weeks of treatment.

Lyme Disease Nosode is effective when used in conjunction with the *simillimum* and is needed to remove the infective obstacle to cure.

---

[143] Peter Alex, *The Homeopathic Treatment of Lyme Disease*, ibid.

Case 17: 39 year old woman

Presenting symptoms:
- Recurring pharyngitis
- Headaches
- Fatigue.

History:
Graves Disease, currently treated with *NeoMercazole*

Her presenting symptoms were thought to be caused by her Graves Disease, despite long term medication with *NeoMercazole*. However, the recurring pharyngitis prompted further investigations, which resulted in the diagnosis of deep gum infection, which had not caused obviously related symptoms. Her gum infection was her obstacle to cure.

Prescription: *Mercurius viv 200c*, one dose once every second day, for three months, which resolved all symptoms. This remedy is specific for deep gum infection.

Deep Gum Infection
Patients with undiagnosed deep gum infections can have no symptoms in the buccal mucosa. Symptoms may be vague and general:
- Fatigue
- Transient raised temperature
- Vague feeling of 'unwellness'
- There may or may not be a raised ESR[144]

In these cases, I recommend *Mercurius viv 200c* once every 2nd day for at least one month. [145]

Case 18: 42 year old man
This man had lifelong fatigue, weakness, disturbed sleep and recurring fevers. He had a history of gum abscesses since he was a child. *Mercurius viv 200c* produced an immediate fever (aggravation). Repeated doses, once every second day, resulted in his complete recovery.

---

[144] Erythrocyte Sedimentation Rate; measures the degree of systemic inflammation
[145] After Dr Parimal Banerji's *Advanced Homeopathy*, Calcutta, India

Appendices

Appendix 1
Pathology Tests & Resources

A positive test result often reveals what needs to be treated and gives confidence to the patient and practitioner. Testing engenders good patient compliance, on account of seeing something 'real' causing their symptoms, which can come as a relief after being told there is nothing that can be done for their illness.

Pathology tests *aid*, but do not *replace* our assessment and diagnosis, as the clinical picture is individual to each patient. While tests provide information about the disease process, they do not tell us which remedy to choose.

Take care not to fall into the trap of addressing pathology and not the patient, as would occur the standard medical approach - the opposite extreme to: "treat the patient not the disease" Which of these approaches is correct? With respect to all leaders and teachers of homeopathy, the homeopathic adage could also be something like: "treat the disease which manifests in *this* patient".

BLOOD TESTS

Full Blood Count

Blood tests have often been done before the patient presents for homeopathic treatment. If not, you may need to check for:

Iron deficiency
In menstruating women and children, especially at 2 years and under with poor appetite or habitual fatigue. Iron deficiency in non-menstruating adults should alert practitioners to the possibility of occult bleeding.[146]

Vitamin B12
B12 deficiency is possible in vegetarians and may be present patients with 'oxidative stress' as found in Autism Spectrum Disorders chronic fatigue, and fibromyalgia.

Gliadin antibodies
Patients with ongoing, unresponsive digestive disease may have coeliac disease and often slip through the gluten allergy screening net. Gliadin antibodies pointing towards coeliac disease are easily identified.

Thyroid Function Tests (TFT's)
Undiagnosed thyroid disease is a common clinical presentation. Patients with unexplained weight gain (or loss), hair loss and palpitations, excessive body

---

[146] "Occult" bleeding refers to bleeding of unknown or hidden origin. This requires further investigation.

heat or chill, anxiety or insomnia should be screened for thyroid disease. Refer to the patient's doctor for testing, or check with home test kits.[147]

Viral titres
A blood test can confirm recent exposure to viruses causing ongoing fatigue and guide homeopathic treatment. Past exposure is a common phenomenon in these tests and is not necessarily diagnostic or helpful.

Common viral pathogens are:
• Epstein Barr virus
• Cytomegalovirus
• Herpes 1 & 2.

Joint pain & swelling
Conditions to suspect in chronic undiagnosed joint pain and swelling:
• Rheumatoid disease:
  o Rheumatoid factor
  o Raised Erythrocyte Sedimentation Rate (ESR)
  o Mycoplasma, Streptococcus, TB[148]
• Dengue fever (Flavivirus), Ross River fever (Ross River Virus)
• Systemic Lupus Erythematosus (SLE): ANA's (anti nuclear antibodies)
• Lyme disease: Borrelia burgdorferi infection

Liver Function Tests (LFT's)
• Conditions with low energy, yellowish complexion, history of alcohol abuse, suspected Hepatitis A, B or C
• Obesity (fatty liver)

Blood: Finger prick tests in clinic

Biocard – instant finger prick tests are available for coeliac disease[149] helicobacter pylori, Candida albicans. These are available online for patients & practitioners.[150]

STOOL TESTS

Complete Digestive Stool Analysis (CDSA)
Used to identify:
Specific parasites, fungi, bacteria, dysbiosis, errors of carbohydrate or protein metabolism.

---

[147] One laboratory which offers home kits can be found at www.healthscopepathology.com.au
[148] See www.roadback.org for extensive information on bacterial involvement in rheumatoid arthritis and other connective tissue disorders
[149] www.coeliactest.com.au
[150] Biocard information is available from Westhead Healthcare 2006. Westhead Group Pty. Ltd. P.O. Box 1133 NEWPORT, NSW 2106. Phone (02) 9999 6518. Fax (02) 9999 6519. Email info@westhead.com.au or www.coeliactest.com.au

Use in unresponsive digestive disease, where gut dysbiosis / intestinal parasites can be an obstacle to cure.[151]

URINE TESTS

Spot iodine test
This is a simple daytime urine test to measure iodine levels. In Australia it is available through doctors on Medicare. Some labs offer this service to natural therapies practitioners.

Iodine levels should be assessed in these conditions:
• Autistic spectrum disorders
• Cystic swelling of endocrine or reproductive tissue, eg goitre, ovarian cysts, fibrocystic breast disease etc
• Developmental delay in children
• Pregnancy (routine screen)
• Thyroid disease.

Urinalysis Test Strips
A urine sample is easy to test in a consultation with a dipstick. All patients should have this simple test done at their first consultation. Positive signs indicate further testing.
Test strips are available from medical suppliers everywhere and easily show:

• Bilirubin (liver disease)
• Glucosuria (diabetes)
• Haematuria (kidney disease)
• Ketones (hyperglycaemia in undiagnosed diabetes, including pregnant women)
• Protein
• Nitrates (urinary tract infection)
• Urine pH: below 6.5 indicates oxidative stress / over acidity and needs correcting

Acid / alkaline levels with pH strips
A simple test that can be done in clinic to measure urinary or saliva pH. Measuring both urine and saliva on several days of the week (by the patient) allows for an accurate assessment of the acid/alkaline status and guides patient compliance.
These can be purchased with bulk discounts at http://www.ph-ion.com/

Indicans
Indicans show the level of pathogenic bacteria (not parasites) in the gut, and is thus a useful marker of gut dysbiosis and leaky gut. The test can be done during the consultation.

---

[151] Gamble, J, *Mastering Homeopathy 2: The Treatment of Irritable Bowel Syndrome,* Karuna Publishing, 2006 available at www.irritablebowelsyndrome.net.au

Intestinal Permeability
IP shows the transit of inappropriate molecules through the gut wall into the bloodstream. (Leaky gut) The test can be done during the consultation.

Heavy Metal Excretion
This urine test that can be done in clinic gives a quick estimation of the current heavy metal load being excreted. The speed and intensity of the colour change from green (normal) to another colour is indicative of a heavy metal presence and gives sound basis for further testing via Hair Tissue Mineral Analysis (see below).
As with all urine tests, you will only see what is being excreted at that time – it is not an accumulative record as is found in hair.

Tests and test kits are available from:
- Great Plains Laboratory

   http://www.greatplainslaboratory.com/home/eng/metals_urine.asp

- Doctor's Data http://www.doctorsdata.com/tests_assessments_info.asp

- Harmonology http://www.harmonology.com.au/

Saliva
Zinc Tally
A subjective assessment of taste response to a liquid zinc challenge gives a quick estimate of the patient's zinc status. Any zinc liquid can provide results, but suppliers will have specific zinc assessment liquids available.

pH strips
Assess the patient's saliva (or urinary) pH easily done in clinic. Measuring both urine and saliva on several days of the week (by the patient) allows for an accurate assessment of the acid/alkaline status. These can be purchased with bulk discounts at http://www.ph-ion.com/

Specialisted Pathology Tests Summary

Cause	Test	Laboratories
Toxic elements[152]: • Cadmium • Copper • Lead • Mercury	Hair Tissue Mineral Analysis (HTMA) – if chronic accumulation suspected General picture of toxic element retention is shown by urine test Blood test – if acute toxicity. Urine test – to check pre and post chelation	Interclinical Laboratories www.interclinical.com.au Healthscope Pathology www.healthscopepathology.com.au Doctors Data Inc www.doctorsdata.com Mediscan www.pointwalterpharmacy.com.au Global Harmony www.harmonology.com.au All pathology labs Most pathology labs
Mineral deficiency	HTMA Blood and urine tests through standard laboratories.	Healthscope Pathology www.healthscopepathology.com.au Doctors Data Inc www.doctorsdata.com Mediscan: www.pointwalterpharmacy.com.au Interclinical Laboratories www.interclinical.com.au Australian Biologics www.australianbiologics.com.au
Coeliac disease	Fingerprick test Blood test.	www.coeliactest.com.au All pathology labs
Intestinal parasites • Helminths • Flukes • Amoebas	3-day stool test with immersion in fixative	Histopath Pathologists www.histopath.com.au Healthscope Pathology www.healthscopepathology.com.au
Chemicals: Organochloride organophosphate pesticides herbicides	Urine and blood	www.testsafe.com.au www.diagnosticinsight.com.au
Lyme Disease	Blood test	Standard laboratories.

---

[152] Other toxic elements not discussed in this book are also revealed in HTMA: aluminium, antimony, arsenic, beryllium, uranium

Appendix 2
Hair Tissue Mineral Analysis

Terminology
These terms are used interchangeably:
- HMA = Hair Mineral Analysis
- HTMA = Hair Tissue Mineral Analysis
- TMA = Tissue Mineral Analysis

Hair analysis is the chemical analysis of a hair sample, used when blood and urine are no longer expected to contain a particular contaminant. It is widely used in forensic toxicology and environmental toxicology.

History of Hair Mineral Analysis
Hair mineral analysis has been used to detect heavy metal toxicity for over 100 years. There are theories of Napoleon dying from arsenic poisoning[153] and Beethoven's deafness being caused by lead poisoning[154]. Hair Mineral Analysis was used in London 100 years ago to determine arsenic poisoning.
While hair mineral analysis is not accepted as a valid form of testing for patients in a medical context, it is used It is an important research tool in archaeology, forensics, epidemiology and environmental research. It is used by the Environment Protection Agency in the USA[155], universities and government agencies around the world to assess nutritional elements and heavy metals. [156], [157] It is also used to monitor patients on programmes for substance abuse.[158]
Hair analysis has become a popular form of testing amongst practitioners treating autism, where deficiency and heavy metal toxicity is common.[159]

Comparing Blood & Hair Testing
Blood reflects the *current* nutritional and toxic element picture only; not *past* or accumulated exposure. Toxins the body is exposed to, stay in blood for short

---

[153] The Death of Napoleon, Cancer or Arsenic? J. Thomas Hindmarsh[1] and John Savory *Clinical Chemistry* http://www.clinchem.org/ 54: 2092-2093, 2008; 10.1373/clinchem.2008.117358
[154] Mai, FM (2006). "Beethoven's terminal illness and death". *The journal of the Royal College of Physicians of Edinburgh* 36 (3): 258–63
[155] Analysis of mercury in hair of EPA region V population. Pellizzari ED, Fernando R, Cramer GM, Meaburn GM, Bangerter K. Research Triangle Institute, Research Triangle Park, North Carolina, 27709, USA. edp@rti.org
[156] Journal of the Forensic Science Society Volume 4, Issue 4, October 1964, Pages 192-199 The Interpretation of the Arsenic Content of Human Hair Hamilton Smith Department of Forensic Medicine, University of Glasgow, Scotland
[157] Agency of Toxic substances and disease registry http://www.atsdr.cdc.gov/HAC/hair_analysis/5.2.html
[158] Pragst F., Balikova M.A.: State of the art in hair analysis for detection of drugs and alcohol abuse; Clinica Chimic Acta 370 2006 17-49.
[159] Lathe, Richard, and Michael Le Page. "Toxic metal clue to autism: a study has revealed startling differences in mercury levels in the hair of autistic and normal children. (This Week)." *New Scientist* 178.2400 (June 21, 2003): 4(2).

periods, sometimes only days, until the body is able to remove them to other tissues, which is what we know as homeostasis. *Think of blood as the body's transit lounge through which all substances briefly pass on their way into the cells.*

Hair
- *Hair* contains minerals and other substances that are incorporated into the hair follicle during its development & locked into the hair shaft as it grows from the scalp.
- Hair provides a more accurate picture of mineral *accumulation* than blood. Minerals are incorporated into the hair as a result of relatively long-term metabolic activity and are therefore more stable than minerals circulating in the blood. Mineral levels can change in the blood over a short period of time, via diet, stress and environment.
- The first 4 centimeters of hair from the scalp reveals tissue levels of minerals and other substances for the previous three months.
- Since hair is an excretory organ, heavy metals can also be detected there if tissue excretion has occurred.

Using Hair Mineral Analysis in a Homeopathic Context
You are faced with an unresponsive patient, and you have applied the *simillimum*, treated the *miasm* and delved deeper. Blood, urine and other tests have been done and you have addressed any abnormalities.

This is the point to search further for an obstacle to cure by gathering more data. In ordering a hair analysis, you are looking for:

- Nutritional abnormalities: deficiency or imbalance: see Chapter 2.
- Toxicity: presence of a heavy metal, or nutrient in excess.

If one or more of these are revealed in the hair analysis results, the treatment direction is clearer. Many natural therapists use hair analysis results to implement an extensive programme of nutritional supplementation, which forms part, or all of, the treatment programme. In a homeopathic context, developing a treatment programme is not the purpose of testing hair. As a homeopath you are looking for an *obstacle to the well-selected remedy from acting*: ie nutritional deficiency, copper accumulation, or heavy metal toxicity. In the case of simple deficiency, which is common, (see Chapter 2 for examples) replacing essential nutrients with supplements can lead to a rapid resolution of a problem, without the need for a potentised remedy.

When to use hair mineral analysis
Having used hair mineral analysis extensively in my practice, there are some conditions that I order at the beginning of treatment. Patients with these conditions almost always reveal nutritional or toxic issues:
- ADD/ADHD
- Autism
- Chronic Fatigue Syndrome
- Crohn's Disease

- Fibromyalgia
- Obstinate Irritable Bowel Syndrome.

Taking a hair sample
When taking a scalp hair sample, the first 4 cms from the scalp is used. This reflects the mineral tissue accumulation and excretion over the previous 3 months. Hair should be untreated with hair colours, dyes etc and should not be shampooed for 3 days before taking the sample to avoid hair shampoo chemicals from affecting results. Take the sample with clean stainless steel scissors.

Hair analyses are available from:
- Australian Biologics www.australianbiologics.com.au
- Doctor's Data (USA) www.doctorsdata.com
- Healthscope Functional Pathology (Melbourne)

  www.healthscopepathology.com.au
- Interclinical Laboratories www.interclinical.com.au
- Point Walter Pharmacy: www.pointwalterpharmacy.com.au

Reading Hair Mineral Analysis Graphs
Understanding hair analysis graphs takes time and practice, but frank deficiencies and toxicities are apparent to any casual observer and provide basic information upon which to base your next prescription.

The following graph shows "Potentially Toxic Elements". Many of these are also essential trace elements: their potential toxicity lies in excessive amounts being retained in the tissues. This is true of any element, even the "good elements" such as calcium.
  However, there are elements which have no place at all in human tissue, that is, any amount is too much. These are the elements we have discussed in this book and described as 'heavy metals'.
These elements are:
- Aluminium (debated whether this is a true heavy metal)
- Antimony
- Arsenic
- Beryllium
- Cadmium
- Lead
- Mercury
- Uranium.

There are two formats used by respective HTMA laboratories. Neither is superior; the choice is a matter of preference. The first format uses a horizontal bar graph. The 'Reference Ranges' show the expected, or 'acceptable' amount of the respective mineral. Once a toxic element accumulates to an extent that it is designated in the first shaded area, this is a significant cautionary amount of the metal, which in many patients will begin to produce toxic symptoms. When it reaches the second shaded area, a significant chronic disease accumulation will have commenced.

Many elements are described as "potentially toxic" if they accumulate past a certain reference point. However, many of these are also nutritional elements. True toxic elements, the "Heavy Metals", have no place in human tissue. These are:

- Aluminium
- Antimony
- Arsenic
- Beryllium
- Cadmium
- Lead
- Mercury
- Uranium.

POTENTIALLY TOXIC ELEMENTS

TOXIC ELEMENTS	RESULT μg/g	REFERENCE RANGE	PERCENTILE 68th	95th
Aluminum	3.0	< 7.0		
Antimony	0.019	< 0.050		
Arsenic	0.019	< 0.060		
Barium	15	< 2.0		
Beryllium	< 0.01	< 0.020		
Bismuth	0.99	< 2.0		
Cadmium	0.046	< 0.050		
Lead	0.20	< 0.60		
Mercury	0.34	< 0.80		
Platinum	0.003	< 0.005		
Thallium	< 0.001	< 0.002		
Thorium	< 0.001	< 0.002		
Uranium	0.002	< 0.060		
Nickel	0.83	< 0.30		
Silver	0.07	< 0.15		
Tin	2.0	< 0.30		
Titanium	0.36	< 0.70		
Total Toxic Representation				

ESSENTIAL AND OTHER ELEMENTS

ELEMENTS	RESULT μg/g	REFERENCE RANGE	PERCENTILE 2.5th	16th	50th	84th	97.5th
Calcium	3050	300- 1200					
Magnesium	310	35- 120					
Sodium	700	20- 250					
Potassium	55	8- 75					
Copper	27	11- 37					
Zinc	190	140- 220					
Manganese	0.13	0.08- 0.60					
Chromium	0.44	0.40- 0.65					
Vanadium	0.023	0.018- 0.065					
Molybdenum	0.010	0.020- 0.050					
Boron	1.3	0.25- 1.5					
Iodine	0.43	0.25- 1.8					
Lithium	0.17	0.007- 0.020					
Phosphorus	143	150- 220					
Selenium	0.80	0.55- 1.1					
Strontium	50	0.50- 7.6					
Sulfur	44300	44000- 50000					
Cobalt	0.015	0.005- 0.040					
Iron	3.5	7.0- 16					
Germanium	0.038	0.030- 0.040					
Rubidium	0.050	0.007- 0.096					
Zirconium	0.058	0.020- 0.42					

SPECIMEN DATA / RATIOS

COMMENTS:

Date Collected: 1/31/2009	Sample Size:	0.195 g	ELEMENTS	RATIOS	EXPECTED RANGE
Date Received: 2/2/2009	Sample Type:	Head	Ca/Mg	9.84	4- 30
Date Completed: 2/4/2009	Hair Color:	Gray	Ca/P	21.3	1- 12
Client Reference:	Treatment:		Na/K	12.7	0.5- 10
Methodology: ICP-MS	Shampoo:	Pantene	Zn/Cu	7.04	4- 20
		V010.08	Zn/Cd	> 999	> 800

Appendix 2: Hair Tissue Mineral Analysis

The alternate table format gives us the vertical bar graphs (see below).

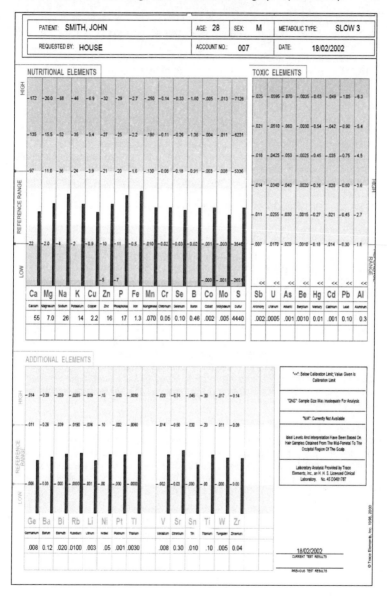

| PATIENT: SMITH, JOHN | AGE: 28 | SEX: M | METABOLIC TYPE: SLOW 3 |
| REQUESTED BY: HOUSE | ACCOUNT NO.: 007 | DATE: 18/02/2002 |

NUTRITIONAL ELEMENTS

Ca	Mg	Na	K	Cu	Zn	P	Fe	Mn	Cr	Se	B	Co	Mo	S
Calcium	Magnesium	Sodium	Potassium	Copper	Zinc	Phosphorus	Iron	Manganese	Chromium	Selenium	Boron	Cobalt	Molybdenum	Sulfur
55	7.0	26	14	2.2	16	17	1.3	.070	0.05	0.10	0.46	.002	.005	4440

TOXIC ELEMENTS

Sb	U	As	Be	Hg	Cd	Pb	Al
Antimony	Uranium	Arsenic	Beryllium	Mercury	Cadmium	Lead	Aluminum
.002	.0005	.001	.0010	0.01	.001	0.10	0.3

ADDITIONAL ELEMENTS

Ge	Ba	Bi	Rb	Li	Ni	Pt	Tl		V	Sr	Sn	Ti	W	Zr
Germanium	Barium	Bismuth	Rubidium	Lithium	Nickel	Platinum	Thallium		Vanadium	Strontium	Tin	Titanium	Tungsten	Zirconium
.008	0.12	.020	.0100	.003	.05	.001	.0030		.008	0.30	.010	.10	.005	0.04

"<<": Below Calibration Limit; Value Given is Calibration Limit

"QNS": Sample Size Was Inadequate For Analysis

"N/A": Currently Not Available

Ideal Levels And Interpretation Have Been Based On Hair Samples Obtained From The Mid-Parietal To The Occipital Region Of The Scalp

Laboratory Analysis Provided by Trace Elements, Inc., an H. H. S. Licensed Clinical Laboratory. No. 45 D0481787

18/02/2002
CURRENT TEST RESULTS

PREVIOUS TEST RESULTS

© Trace Elements, Inc. 1998, 2000

173

Treatment guided by hair tissue mineral analysis:

Nutritional elements

In this book we have consistently used the second format for the sake of consistency. In this second format table, the top left box gives the essential minerals, starting from the most important to the least important, left to right. The ideal level is in the centre of the unshaded area called 'Reference Range'.

Additional elements

The bottom box shows the trace elements. These are the micro particles, which assist in maintaining cell health. One can live without many of these minerals, but optimum health is achieved by making sure we have all of them in our tissue. Most people will commonly lack one or more of these additional elements. Some of them will result in disease if they are deficient, such as iodine, which is discussed below. Others will generate a tendency, or a disease potential, if deficient, such as lithium, a deficiency of which will engender a tendency towards anxiety.

Toxic elements

The upper box on the right shows the toxic elements. These elements are inimical to life. Any amount of either element is too much. Small amounts of these elements may pass through us every day: this is a normal consequence of living in the modern world. These transient amounts can be found in the unshaded section box, called 'Reference Range'. If we do not efficiently excrete them and they accumulate in our tissues, this underpins the chronic disease process, forming as it does an obstacle to cure. Once a toxic element has accumulated to such an extent that it is indicated in the firsr shaded area, this represents a cautionary amount, which may have begun producing disease symptoms. If it has accumulated into the higher, deep shaded area, this is a significant amount of the toxic element, which will in most cases be producing observable chronic symptoms. Many of the cases examples in this book show a toxic burden off the graph entirely: this represents a significant danger to health.

Comparing both types of graph, you can see that the horizontal graph lists more toxic elements than the vertical graph. The reason for this is that the former lists "potential toxic elements". Many of these are also trace elements, which have nutritional value and only become toxic when they are in excess. It is these eight toxic elements below which have no nutritional, value and ought not to be found in human tissue at all.

- Aluminium
- Antimony
- Arsenic
- Beryllium
- Cadmium
- Lead
- Mercury
- Uranium

The most common mineral found in excess in humans is copper: see Ch 5.

174

Appendix 3
Treatment Summaries: How to Remove Obstacles to Cure

Obstacle	Treatment
All nutritive mineral deficiencies	Give bio-available mineral supplement. Ensure nutrition is optimal. Ensure no digestive issues affecting ability to absorb nutrients. Ensure there are no toxic antagonists to the mineral (eg lead undermines calcium absorption)
Toxic elements: cadmium	Cadmium chelate: 1 dose every 2nd day. Zinc: 30mg elemental zinc per day
Toxic element: excess copper	Copper chelate: 1 dose every 2nd day. Zinc: 30mg elemental zinc per day
Toxic element: lead	Lead Chelate: 1 dose every 2nd day. Ensure daily amounts of calcium and iron to provide antagonistic activity
Toxic element: mercury	Mercury chelate: 1 dose every 2nd day. Zinc: 30mg elemental zinc daily. Selenium: 250mcg daily (caution taking selenium for long periods)
Vaccine sequelae	Vaccine 30c – 2 doses week 1. Vaccine 200c – 2 doses week 2. Vaccine 1M – 2 doses week 3. Vaccine 10M – 2 doses week 4.
Oral Contraceptive Pill	Folliculinum 30c: 1 dose every 2nd day for two weeks.
Antibiotic sequelae	Penicillin or Amoxicillin 30c: 1 dose every 2nd day for two weeks. Candida treatment if needed[160]
Confused iatrogenic drug pictures	Camphor 200c – 1 dose every 2nd day for 2 to 8 weeks.
Pesticide, Herbicide & Fungicide exposure	Pesticide, Herbicide & Fungicide Protocol 200c/3; 30c/3; 16c/3; 16c/3; 30c/3; 200c/3
Industrial Chemicals (including hydrocarbons) exposure	Industrial Chemicals Protocol 200c/3; 30c/3: 16c/3; 16c/3; 30c/3; 200c/3
Xenoestrogen accumulation	Xenoestrogen Protocol 200/3; 30c/3; 16c/3; 16c/3; 30c/3; 200c/3 + zinc supplement if needed
Electro-magnetic radiation	Radium Bromide 200c or X-ray 200c (throw out the mobile phone)
Deep Gum infection	Mercurius vivus 200c: 1 dose every 2nd day

---

[160] Gamble, J, *Mastering Homeopathy 2: The Treatment of Irritable Bowel Syndrome*, Karuna Publishing, 2006, p 61

Obstacle	Treatment
Lyme disease	Lyme disease nosode 30c on alternate days with remedy of choice (Rhus tox, Gelsemium, etc)
Post-viral syndromes	Coxsackievirus nosode or Cytomegalovirus nosode on alternate days with remedy of choice
Intestinal parasites	Cina 200c; Stannum 200c; Teucrium 200c; Trichinose nosode 30c
Mosquito-born diseases	Give nosode of the relevant disease on alternate days to remedy of choice

Appendix 4
Contents of the Chemical Protocols

Protocol 1 (Pesticides, Herbicides and Fungicides)

The chemicals in this list are contained in Protocol 1 (see Chapter 6).

Trade Name or Chemical	Use	Health Effects
Cuprox	Antifouling agent Copper oxide	Possible endocrine disruptor
Carboryl	Pesticide Banned in Australia 2007 but still available: Hortico Tomato Dust Yates Tomato Gun Bernard Flea Powder	Carcinogen
Benomyl	Fungicide	Endocrine disruptor Carcinogen
2.4.D	Herbicide, ingredient in Agent Orange	Carcinogen; still used in aerial spraying in Australia(2010)
Aldicarb	Pesticide	Cholinesterase inhibitor
Asulam	Herbicide	Still in use
10 80	Poison used to kill introduced animals eg rabbits	Still in use
Amitrole	Weedkiller	Still in use; carcinogen
Permethrin	Pyrethroid Pesticide	Still in use
2,4,5,T	Organochloride herbicide; ingredient in Agent Orange	2,3,7,8-tetrachlorodibenzo-p-dioxin (TCDD) is produced as byproduct in manufacturing, which is carcinogenic
Dicamba	Organochloride weedkiller	Reproductive toxin
Dicophane	DDT Pesticide	
DDT	Organhochloride pesticide	Carcinogen; reproductive & developmental toxin; known to cause diabetes
Dichlorvos	Cockroach and flea insecticide, including flea collars	Cholinesterase inhibitor
Diazinon	Pesticide	Cholinesterase inhibitor; banned
Dursban	Pesticide	Cholinesterase inhibitor; banned
Dieldrin		
Copper sulphate	Mould and algae	Endocrine; liver; carcinogen; reproductive disruptor
Chlordane	Organochloride pesticide	Carcinogenic: prostate Ca; leukaemia
Cyanide	Acute toxicity	
Cypermethrin	Insecticide Found in RAID cockroach killer.	Possible carcinogen and endocrine disruptor. Excessive exposure: nausea, headache, muscle weakness, salivation, shortness of breath and seizures
Lindane		
Phosmet	Organophosphate insecticide	Cholinesterase inhib, carcinogen

177

Trade Name or Chemical	Use	Health Effects
Heptachlor	Organophosphate insecticide	
Azinphos Methyl	Organophosphate insecticide	Cholinesterase inhibitor
Omethoate	Organophospate insecticide	Cholinesterase inhibitor
DichloFluanid	Wood preservative, fungicide	Endocrine disruptor and others
Endosulfan	Insecticide	Endocrine disruptor;
Methyl 2,3,4 D-Phenothrin Tetramethrin	Pyrethroid insecticide	
Fenarimol	Fungicide	Endocrine disruptor
Paraquat	Herbicide	Carcinogen; Cholinesterase inhibitor; pot sprayed with in then smoked: 'Paraqat Pot'; Parkinsons Disease
Metiram	Fungicide	Carcinogen and endocrine reproductive disruptor
Paraquat Diquat	Herbicide	As for paraquat
Pyrethrum	Pesticide from chrysanthemum family	
Glyphosate N	Herbicide	Toxicity not known
Maldison	Organophosphate pesticide (fleas, lice)	Potential carcinogen
MCPA	Phenoxy group herbicide	Unknown
Maneb		Carcinogen, reproductive, endocrine; Parkinsons disease
Methyl Bromide (bromomethane)	Pesticide organobromine Fire suppressant Electricity substations	Restricted. Neurological & respiratory systems.
Famphur	Organophosphate	Cholinesterase inhibitor
Thiram	Fungicide	Cholinesterase; reproductive disruptor
Mecoprop MCPA	Hormone type phenoxy herbicide	Carcinogen
Sulphur		
Simazine	Triazine class herbicide used in swimming pools	Hormone disruptor
Fluazinam	Fungicide	Possible carcinogen
Triflorine	Fungicide	Unknown
Triflorine acephaye		
Simazine	Herbicide (triazine) used in swimming pools.	Unknown; Reproductive and endocrine
Vinclozolin	Fungicide	Carcinogen; endocrine and reproductive
Methiocarb	Pesticide (carbamate)	Cholinesterase inhibitor
Hydrogen cyanamide	Inorganic herbicide	Acute toxicity; poss carcinogen
Glyphosate trimesium	Phosphonglycine herbicide	Acute toxicity only
Fonofos	Organophosphate pesticide	Banned. Cholinesterase inhibitor.
Chloro Thalonil	Fungicide	Carcinogen
Clopyralid	Pyridiniccarboloxinic acid herbicide	Unknown
Chlorpyriphos	Organophosphate herbicide	Cholinesterase inhibitor
Bromacil diuren	Herbicide	Suspected carcinogen & endocrine disruptor

Trade Name or Chemical	Use	Health Effects
Metsulfuron	Urea herbicide	Unknown
Acephate	Organophosphate insecticide	Cholinesterase inhibitor
Triclopyr	Chloropyridynal herbicide	Unknown
Bromofenoxin	Pesticide Similar to 2,4-D	
Tau Fluvalinate	Pyrethroid insecticide	Developmental or reproductive toxin
Picloram 2,4,D	Pyridine family pesticide	
Phorate	Organophosphate pesticide	Cholinesterase inhibitor
Octhilinone	Fungicide	Unknown
Terbufos	Organophosphate pesticide	Cholinesterase inhibitor
MCPB	Herbicide chlorophenoxy acid	Possible carcinogen
Methomyl	N-Methyl Carbamatye insecticide	Cholinesterase inhibitor; possible endocrine disruptor
Napthyl acetic acid	Plant hormone used as fertilizer	Chronic health effects unknown
Copper oxine B 3	Fungicide	None known (apart from xenoestrogenic)
Copper naphthenate B 3	Fungicide, animal repellant, wood preservative	Not known (apart from xenoestrogen)
Chlorothalon thiophanate	Fungicide	Unknown
Cca concentrate	Fungicide: arsenic, copper and hexavalent chromiun	
Carbendazim	Fungicide	Hormonal disruptor, carcinogen, reproductive and mutagenic effects
Acetochlor	Herbicide chloroacetanilide	Carcinogen
Hexachlor-benzene	Organochloride Chlorocarbon fungicide	Carcinogen
Haloxyfop	Aryloxyphenoxy propionic acid	Unknown
Glyphosate r glL	Phosphonoglycine	Unknown
Furalaxyl	Fungicide	Unknown
Fipronil propanol	Insecticide	Frontline for cats, / agriculture Toxicity unknown
Fenitrothion	Organophosphate herbicide	Cholinesterase inhibitor
Dimethoate	Organophosphae insecticide	Cholinesterase inhibitor; teratogenic, carcinogenic, reproductive
Diflu-benzuron	Insecticide	Unknown
Cyproconazollodocarb	Pesticide	Unknown
Oxadiazon	Herbicine	Carcinogen; developmental / reproductive toxin
Oryzalin	Herbicine	Carcinogen, reproductive toxin
Ortho dichlo benzene	Herbicide organic halogen	Unknown
Mctolachlor	Herbicide chloroacetanilide	Suspected carcinogen, suspected endocrine disruptor
Metalaxyl manozeb	Fungicide	Unknown
Imidazole prochloraz	Fungicide	Suspected carcinogen and endocrine disruptor
Quintozene	Agricultural fungicide – contains dioxin	Potential carcinogen

Trade Name or Chemical	Use	Health Effects
Propoxur	Carbamate pesticide	Carcinogen; Cholinesterase inhibitor
Pirimiphos methyl	Organophosphate pesticide	Carcinogen; Cholinesterase inhibitor
Picloram triclopyr	Herbicide	
Permethrin pyrethrum	Pyrethrum is gradually replacing the organophosphates and organochlorides	
Permethrin		
Pentachlorphenol (PCP)	Organochloride pesticide	Carcinogen
Tolclofos methyl	Organophosphate pesticide	Cholinesterase inhibitor
Temephos	Organophosphate pesticide	Cholinesterase inhibitor
Camphechlor	Organochloride pesticide	
Coumaphos	Organophosphate	Cholinesterase inhibitor
Cuprofezin	Insecticide	Possible carcinogen
Bendiocarb	Carbamate insectidice	
2-4-D butyl ester	Chlorophenoxy herbicide	Possible carcinogen
2-4-D dicamba	Benzoic herbicide	Possible teratogen
Azinphos-met cahptan	Pesticide	
Atrazine	Triazine herbicide	
Azocyclotin	Organotin herbicide	Suspected endocrine disruptor
Diazinon ethyl brom	organophosphate	Cholinesterase inhibitor
diquat	Herbicide	Unknown
Dienochlor	Organochloride	Unknown
Dodine	Fungicide	Unknown
D-Phenothrin	Insecticide	Suspected endocrine disruptor
Copper oxychloride	Fungicide	Endocrine disruptor
Cyromazine	Triazine insecticide	Unknown
Cupric hydroxide	Fungicide	Endocrine disruptor; Wilson's disease
Clofentezine	Tetrazine insecticide	Endocrine disruptor
Chlorothal thiophanate	Pesticide	Unknown
Iprodione	Fungicide	Carcinogen
Glufosinate ammonium	Herbicide	Neurotoxic; teratogenic (birth defects)
Fosetyl aluminium	Fungicide	Unknown
Flusilazole	Fungicide	Unknown
Fenpyroximat	Insecticide	Unknown
Diuron terbuthylazi	Hormone triazine herbicide	Unknown
Diazinon permethrin	Insecticide DDT based product.	Neurotoxin.
Dioxin	Chemical byproducts (incl some pesticides like agent orange	Carcinogen
Deltamethrin	Pyrethroid insecticide	Unknown
Diful benzuron	Insecticide growth regulator	
Parathion	Organophosphate pescticide	Carcinogen
Picloram	Pyridine herbicide	Suspected endocrine disruptor

Appendix 4: Chemical Protocols

Trade Name or Chemical	Use	Health Effects
PendiMethanlin	Herbicide 2,6-Dinitroaniline	Suspected endocrine disruptor
Propargite	Insecticide	Carcinogen; reproductive toxin
Myclobutanil	Fungicide	Reproductive toxin, suspected endocrine disruptor
Metiram-Nitr Isopropyl	Carbamate fungicide	Carcinogen; reproductive toxin
Myclobutanil	Fungicide	Reproductive toxin, suspected endocrine disruptor
Isoguard 50	Herbicide	
Zineb	Fungicide	Carcinogen, reproductive and teratogenic
Captan	FUNGICIDE	Carcinogen
Triadimefon	Fungicide	Reproductive toxin; suspected carcinogen and endocrine disruptor
Terbumeton termuthylazi	Triazine herbicide	Unknown
Terbu thylazine	Herbicide	
Trichlorton	Organophosphate	
Tebu conazole	Fungicide	
Trichlor ethane	DDT	As above
P.C.P.	PENTACHLOROPHENOL insecticide	

Protocol 2: Industrial Chemicals
The chemicals in this list are contained in Protocol 2 (see Chapter 6).

Trade Name or Chemical	Use	Health Effects
Methyl 2,3,4	Bio ingredient in some foods and cosmetics	
Butoxy ethanol	Solvent found in paint, ink, liquid soap, cosmetics, white board	Contact sensivitity. Reproductive toxin and haemolytic anaemia in rats
Benzene	Petroleum product from coal tar; cigarettes, coke ovens, petroleum.	Leukaemia; affects the blood forming cells in the bone marrow resulting in anaemia
Bacillus thur kurstak	Biological insecticide – micro-organism form toxic crystals similar to endotoxin	
Etridiazole xylene	Fungicide	Unknown
Paint stripper PS Paint stripper kS Paint stripper RS		
Ortho Dichlo Benzene		
Hydrepoxy	Industrial adhesive	Possible endocrine and reproductive toxin, sensitivity reactions
Hydrepoxy 3200		
Rhodamine B acetic acid	Fluorescent dye	Carcinogen

181

Appendix 4: Chemical Protocols

Trade Name or Chemical	Use	Health Effects
Petrol UL 98 octane		
Petrol UL 91 octane		
Xylene 100 thinners		Respiratory, neurological, toxic in large doses
Xylene	"	"
White spirits	Hydrocarbon used in paint, etc	Neurological sx
Universal paint thinner		
Toluene	Benzene derived hydrocarbon thinner	
Thinners		
Solvent A		
Dioxin	Chemical byproducts (incl some pesticides like agent orange)	Carcinogen
PCB (polychlorinated biphenol)	POP found in coolants, transformers, fire retardants, old plasticizers	Carcinogenic; dioxins
Polyvinyl chloride	Vinyl polymer plastic in clothing, upholstery, flooring	

Protocol 3: Xenoestrogens
The chemicals in this list are contained in Protocol 3 (see Chapter 6).

Trade Name or Chemical	Use	Health Effects
Synthetic oestrogen (Folliculinum)	Homeopathically potentised oestrogen	All xenoestrogens
Polyvinyl Chloride	Vinyl polymer plastic in clothing, upholstery, flooring	"
Mixed hard and soft plastics	Giving a variety of food grade and other (hard) plastics containing phthalates and bisphenol A	"
PCB (polychlorinated biphenol)	POP found in coolants, transformers, fire retardants, plasticizers, paints	Carcinogenic; dioxins
Erythrosine E127 (FD&C Red No 3)	Food colouring	Xenoestrogens
Parabens	Body lotions	"
Butilated Hydroan E320	Food preservative	"
Phenol	Cosmetics, hair dyes, plastic manufacturing	"

182

References and Bibliography

Homeopathy

Allen, Dr H, *Materia Medica of the Nosodes, (1910)*

Alex, Peter, *The Homeopathic Treatment of Lyme Disease*, HomeopathyWest Publishing, 2006

Boericke, *Homoeopathic Materia Medica,* 1st British ed, Homoeopathic Books Service, Kent, UK, 1987

Cole, J & Dyson, R, *Classical Homeopathy Revisited*, UK, after the work of Pritnam Singh.

J Compton-Burnett, *Vaccinosis and its Cure by Thuja* (1897) (B Jain imprint)

Elmiger, Dr J, *Rediscovering Real Medicine: New Horizons in Homeopathy*, Vega, London, 2001

Gamble, J, *Mastering Homeopathy,* Karuna Publishing, 2004; *Mastering Homeopathy 2: The Treatment of Irritable Bowel Syndrome*, Karuna Publishing, 2006

Hahnemann, Dr S, *Organon of Medicine,*5th & 6th *eds,* translated by R Dudgeon, B Jain Publishers, New Delhi, 1990 ed.

Hahnemann, Dr S, *Materia Medica Pura,* (1811-1821) (B. Jain Publishers reprint)

Murphy, R, *Homeopathic Medical Repertory,* Hahnemann Academy of North America, 1993

Ramakrishnan, Dr A, *A Homeopathic Approach to Cancer,* Quality Medical Publishing Inc, Missouri, 2001

Swayne, J, *International Dictionary of Homeopathy,* Churchill Livingstone, 2000

Tumminello, P, *Twelve Jewels,* The Medicine Way, Sydney, 2005; *The Child's Mind and Behaviour,* The Medicine Way, Sydney, 2001

Websites:
Tinus Smits: http://www.post-vaccination-syndrome.com/3890/treatment.aspx

Iatrogenesis

Golden, Isaac, *Vaccine Damaged Children: Treatment, Prevention, Reasons,* Isaac Golden Publications, Australia

Halverson, Dr Richard, *The Truth About Vaccines: How We are Used as Guinea Pigs Without Knowing it,* Gibson Square, London, 2007

Wakefield, Andrew, *Callous Disregard,* Slyhorse Publishing, USA, 2010

Infection

Allen, W, *The War on Bugs*, ISBN-13: 978-1933392462

Ginsburg, J, 'Coughs and Sneezes Spread Diseases', New Scientist, 2472, Nov 2004.

Scammell, H *New Arthritis Breakthrough: the Road Back,* Evans, USA, 1998

Websites & Journals:

http://www.adhd.com.au/PANDAS.htm

http://www.mayoclinic.com/health/blastocystis-hominis/DS00791

http://emedicine.medscape.com/article/997239-overview

Insel, Thomas, 'Microbes and Mental Illness'
http://www.nimh.nih.gov/about/director/2010/microbes-and-mental-illness.shtml

Toxic Chemicals

Rapp, Dr D, *Our Toxic World, A Wake-Up Call,* Environmental Medical Research Foundation, NY, 2004

Reuben, S, *Reducing Environmental Cancer Risk: What we can do Now,* The President's Cancer Panel, USA Dept of Health and Human Services, 2010.

Smith, R, & Lourie, B, *Slow Death by Rubber Duck: How the Toxic Chemistry of Everyday Life Affects our Health,* University of Queensland Press, 2009

Websites and Journals:

ABC Rural: http://www.abc.net.au/rural/content/2006/s1712479.htm

Allmyr, M, "Triclosan in Plasma and Milk from Swedish Nursing Mothers and Their Exposure via Personal Care Products", Science of the Total Environment 372, no 1 (2006): 87-93

Buterin T, Koch C, Naegeli H (August 2006). "Convergent transcriptional profiles induced by endogenous estrogen and distinct xenoestrogens in breast cancer cells". *Carcinogenesis* 27 (8): 1567–78. doi:10.1093/carcin/bgi339. PMID 16474171

Colborn, T, Dumanski, D and Peterso Myres, J, *Our Stolen Future: Are We Threatening our Fertility, Intelligence and Survival?* Penguin Books, NY, 1996

Cox, C, "2,4-D Toxicology: Part 2", Journal of Pesticide Reform 19, no 2, Summer 1999.

Cox, C, "Carbaryl", Journal of Pesticide Reform, Spring 1993: 13 (1), Northwest Coalition for Alternatives to Pesticides, Eugene:

http://panna.igc.org/resources/pestis/PESTIS.1996.18.html

Darbre PD (March 2006). "Environmental oestrogens, cosmetics and breast cancer" *Best Pract. Res. Clin. Endocrinol. Metab.* 20 (1): 121–43. doi:10.1016/j.beem.2005.09.007. PMID 16522524.

Darbre PD, Aljarrah A, Miller WR, Coldham NG, Sauer MJ, Pope GS (2004). "Concentrations of parabens in human breast tumours" *J Appl Toxicol* 24 (1): 5–13. doi:10.1002/jat.958. PMID 14745841

Foran, C, et al, "Developmental Evaluation of a Potential Non-steroidal Estrogen: Triclosan", Marine Environmental Research 50 (2000): 153-56

http://www.atsdr.cdc.gov/csem/benzene/physiologic_effects.html

http://www.epa.gov/ttn/atw/hlthef/phenylen.html

http://www.epa.gov/ttn/atw/hlthef/phenylen.html

http://www.smh.com.au/environment/study-puts-pesticides-safety-in-spotlight-once-again-20090920-fwsw.html

Mol Cancer Ther May 2002,1; 515 http://mct.aacrjournals.org/content/1/7/515.full

Pugazhendhi D, Sadler A J, Darbre PD (2007). "Comparison of the global gene expression profiles produced by methylparaben, n-butylparaben and 17beta-oestradiol in MCF7 human breast cancer cells" *J Appl Toxicol* 27 (1): 67–77. doi:10.1002/jat.1200. PMID 17121429.

Sherman, J M, MD, *Chemical Exposure and Disease: Diagnostic and Investigative Techniques,* 1994, Princeton Scientific Publishing;

Steinman, D & Wisner, R, *Living Health in a Toxic World,* Berkley Publishing Group, New York, NY, 1995

Vidaeff AC, Sever LE (2005). "In utero exposure to environmental estrogens and male reproductive health: a systematic review of biological and epidemiologic evidence". *Reprod. Toxicol.* 20 (1): 5–20.

www.pesticideinfo.org

Mineral Deficiency, Nutrition and Heavy Metals

Gaitan, E, 'Goitrogens in Food and Water', *Annual Review of Nutrition,* 1990; 10: 21-39

Groff, J, & Gropper, S, *Advanced Nutrition and Human Metabolism,* 3rd ed, Wadsworth/Thompson Learning, USA, 2000

Lynch, S, 'Interaction of Iron with other Nutrients', *Nutrition Review,* 1997; 55(4)

Nutrition Almanac 1989 McGraw Hill Book Co

Osieki, H, *Nutrients in Profile,* Bioconcepts Publishing 2nd ed

Saris, J & Wardle, J, eds, *Clinical Naturopathy, An Evidence-Based Guide to Practice,* Churchill Livingstone, Sydney 2010

Shils, M, et al, *Modern Nutrition in Health and Disease,* Lippincott Williams & Wilkins, 2006

Sichel, M, *How to Repair Children Damaged by Mercury, Medicine and Politics,* Fountaindale Books, Sydney, 2007

Sichel, M, *The Sichel Protocol,* Bookbound Publishing, Ourimbah, Australia, 2007

Tabrizian, Dr Igor, *Practitioner's Guide to Reading a Tissue Mineral Analysis,* NRS Publications, ISBN 0975692046

Watts, David, *Trace Elements and Other Essential Nutrients,* 4th Ed, Writer's Block, Texas, 2003

Ziegler, E & Filer, J, eds, *Present Knowledge in Nutrition,* 7th ed, ILSI Press, Washington, 1996

Websites and Journals:

Sambrook, P, "Corticosteroid osteoporosis" Best Pract Res Clin Rheumatol. 2001 Jul; 15(3): 401-13. http://www.ncbi.nlm.nih.gov/pubmed/11485337

Cadmium:

University of Pittsburgh Medical Centre:
http://www.upmc.com/healthatoz/pages/healthlibrary.aspx?chunkiid=120796

http://www.kanazawa-med.ac.jp/~pubhealt/cadmium2/itaiitai-e/itai01.html

Calcium:

Research: Effect of calcium supplements on risk of myocardial infarction and cardiovascular events: meta-analysis http://www.bmj.com/cgi/content/full/341/jul29_1/c3691

Copper:

Bremner, I, 'Manifestations of Copper Excess' *American Journal of Clinical Nutrition,* Vol 67, 1069S-1073S

Gaetke, L, et al, Copper Toxicity, Oxidative Stress and Antioxidant Nutrients, *Toxicology,* 2003 doi:10.1016/j.physletb.2003.10.071

Kitzberger, R, et al, 'Wilson Disease', *Metabolic Brain Disease* 2005, Dec; 20(4), 295-302

Lead:

Rossi, E (1 May 2008). "Low level environmental lead exposure - a continuing challenge" (Free full text). *The Clinical Biochemist. Reviews / Australian Association of Clinical Biochemists* **29** (2): 63–70. ISSN 0159-8090

Pearce, J. M. S. (2007). "Burton's line in lead poisoning". *European neurology* **57** (2): 118–119.

Mercury:

US Centre for Disease Control: "Mercury and Vaccines (Thiomersal)"
http://www.cdc.gov/vaccinesafety/concerns/thiomersal.htm

Zinc:

www.usyd.edu.au/agric/acpa/people/budi/selenium.htm

Audio interviews

Interview by Dr Stanley Morfeith with Dr Jorge Flechas on the BENEFITS OF IODIINE

Index

Index

Index

Death from, 118
Guillain-Barre Syndrome, 118
Gelsemium, 132, 156
Gliadin antibody test, 163
Globus hystericum, 16
Glyphosate, 146
Goiter, 17
Gum infection, 161

Hahnemann – see also *Organon*, 21,
Hair Tissue Mineral Analysis, 168-74
Halverson, R, 116
Hashimoto's thyroiditis, 106
Headache, 42
Heavy metal urine test, 166
Hepar sulph, 113, 128, 155
Hepatitis C, 119
Heptachlor, 97, 101, 102
    Carcinogen, 101
    Hormone disruptor, 101
Herpes zoster, 20
Hexachlorobenzene, 96, 98
    Carcinogen, 101
    Hormone disruptor, 101
Hexachlorophene, 102
Homeostasis, 55
Hormone replacement therapy, side
effects, 115
Hydrocarbons toxicity 100-101
    2-4-5-T. 101, 102
    Benzene, 100
    Bone marrow cancer, 100
    Developmental delay, 100
    Lymphoma from, 101
    Nervous system damage, 100
    Toluene, 100
    Toxic effect, 101
    Xylene, 100
Hypothyroid, 17, 23
    Iodine, and, 28
    Iron, and, 29-30
    Selenium, and 39

Iatrogenesis, definition, 113
Ignatia, 16
In vitro, 55
Indicans test, 165
Infertility, 37
Influenza vaccination, 116
Insomnia, 42
Intestinal permeability test, 166
Iodine test, 165
Itai-itai disease, 68
Kidney reflux, 155

Lead toxicity, 79-83
    Abdominal pain in, 80

Aggression in, 79
Anaemia, in, 80
Astrocytoma in, 81
Bone pain in, 80
Caravaggio, 79
Children, and, 80
Chronic Fatigue Syndrome
83,131-6
    Constipation, in 80, 82
    Fatigue in, 79-80, 82, 83, 131-136
    Fibromyalgia in, 80, 82
    Headache in, 79-80, 82
    Hyperkinetic in, 79
    Insomnia, in, 83
    Memory loss in, 79-80
    Muscle pain in, 79
    Muscle weakness in, 80
    Provings of, 80
    Removal of, 80-81
    Roman empire, 79
    Sources of, 79-80
Lindane, 97-98, 102, 106
    Carcinogen, 101
    Hormone disruptor, 101
    Lice treatment, for 98
    Lymphoma, from, 98
Liver drainage, 107
Lycopodium, 155
Lyme disease, 158-160

Macular degeneration, 37
Magnetis Polis Ambo, 122
MCPA, 146
MMR vaccination, 117, 119
Malathion, 97
Mancozeb, 146
Memory loss, 42
Meniere's disease, 139
Meningococcal vaccination, 117
Mental illness, 37
Mercury toxicity, 84-88
    'foggy head' in, 84-85
    Amalgams, and, 86
    Anxiety in, 85
    Autism in, 84-86
    Candida in, 88
    Colitis, in 84
    Concentration difficulty in, 84
    Dermatitis in, 84-85
    Fatigue in, 84-85, 88
    Gingivitis in, 85
    Headaches in, 85
    Intestinal parasites in, 85, 88
    Intestinal permeability in, 84-85
    Irritable bowel syndrome in, 85,
88-9
    Leaky gut in, 87

189

Index

Index

Acknowledgements

Interclinical Laboratories, Sydney, gave permission to reproduce examples of the Hair Tissue Mineral Analyses.

Doctors' Data, USA, for permission to reprint the HTMA on p 172.